Oliver Klatt

Reiki Systems of the World

One Heart—Many Beats

With contributions by Don Alexander, Phyllis Lei Furumoto,
Walter Lübeck, Paul David Mitchell, Frank Arjava Petter,
William Lee Rand, and others

Translated by Christine M. Grimm

LOTUS PRESS · SHANGRI-LA

First English Edition 2006
© by Lotus Press
P. O. Box 325, Twin Lakes, WI 53181, USA
website: www.lotuspress.com
email: lotuspress@lotuspress.com
The Shangri-La Series is published in cooperation
with Schneelöwe Verlagsberatung, Federal Republic of Germany
© 2004 by Windpferd Verlagsgesellschaft mbH, Aitrang, Germany
All rights reserved
Translated by Christine M. Grimm
Cover layout: Peter Krafft Designagentur, Bad Krozingen, Germany
Interior illustrations: Janine Warmbier, based on photos representing Annett Landmann and also Simone von Mach
ISBN-13: 978-0-914955-79-5
ISBN-10: 0-914955-79-9
Library of Congress Control Number: 2005937340

Printed in USA

Table of Contents

Preface

This book is the result of my many years of involvement with the various forms of the Usui System of Reiki, as well as with the history of this simple and effective method of healing. Originally from Japan, the Usui System of Reiki reached the United States in the middle of 20th century. From here, it ultimately spread throughout the world. Several million people throughout the world now practice the Usui System of Reiki, and this number increases every day. This makes Reiki, in addition to yoga, one of the most widespread spiritual traditions in the world.

This book reveals the entire variety of the Usui System of Reiki. It clearly shows both the commonalities and the differences of the various styles and forms, as well as the impressive history of the system that has been summarized in its entirety in one book for the first time. All of the information, facts, commentaries, and practical exercises come from experienced Reiki Masters and teachers, including many well-known personalities of the worldwide Reiki scene who have been practicing the Usui System of Reiki for many years.

For many of decades, the legendary story according to Mrs. Takata (see pg. 9 ff.) was the only source for anyone interested in the history of the Usui System. This book starts at a different place: It compiles all of the important contents and facts that show the development of the system and its variety from today's standpoint. Of course, this is also not the "ultimate truth." However—and this is my hope—this book can perhaps contribute to Reiki Masters and practitioners becoming increasingly at peace with the roots of the system that they practice and teach today. In addition, this book will help readers interested in Reiki to acquire a good overview of the various forms of the Usui System and make a well-informed choice based on this foundation.

I would like to thank all those who have contributed to this book, who have helped me compile the information, and who have examined the completed texts for their accuracy.

This book is intended to be a contribution to the current developments within the worldwide Reiki scene, which is increasingly characterized by mutual tolerance and appreciation. That such a colorful variety of Reiki Masters and teachers as Phyllis Lei Furumoto, Frank Arjava Petter, Walter Lübeck, Don Alexander, William Lee Rand and Tanmaya Honervogt have contributed to this book fills me with joy and once again highlights the mutual spirit of this work, which is directed at the hearts and minds of the readers beyond any boundaries.

Oliver Klatt

Prolog
The Legend

At the end of the 19th Century, Dr. Mikao Usui, a Christian priest, taught Religious Studies at a small university in the city of Kyoto. One day after class, two of his students came to him and asked: "You have told us stories from the Bible and how Jesus healed the sick by laying his hands on them. Can you also tell us how Jesus did that?" Dr. Usui did not have an answer to this question. This preoccupied him so much that he ended his work as a teacher soon thereafter and set out to find an answer to this question.

His path first led him to America, where he began studying Comparative Religion at a large university. However, this did not get him any further. So he soon returned to Asia, traveled through various countries, and finally came back to Japan. During his journeys he had discovered that not only Jesus but also Buddha had possessed the ability of healing through the laying on of hands. Dr. Usui retreated to a Buddhist monastery to meditate and get closer to answering his question in this way. One day, he discovered scrolls in the library of the monastery that contained a description of how Buddha had healed with his hands. Dr. Usui's search had ended: He now had the knowledge about how to heal by laying on hands. Yet, what he still lacked was the power to translate this knowledge into reality. He conferred with the abbot of the monastery, and both agreed that it would be best for Dr. Usui to retreat into the mountains, fasting and meditating there for 21 days in order to achieve practical access to the knowledge he had found.

Dr. Usui soon set off for the mountains. There he found a beautiful little spot, directly in front of a waterfall, where he settled down. On the first day, he lined up 21 stones in front of himself. Every day he threw one of them away. This helped him keep track of the time that he was spending up there. Nothing happened for a very long time, and Dr. Usui already wanted to give up. Yet, during the very last night he perceived a light on the horizon that slowly came closer and moved directly toward him. When it finally hit his head, he felt opened and completely free. He saw symbols in light bubbles rising before him, and he was spontaneously given the knowledge of Reiki.

Now that he had reached his goal, he made his way back down into the valley the next day. After the long hours of sitting, he was still unaccustomed to walking and stubbed a toe on a stone. He immediately placed both hands on the painful spot and the pain soon went away. Somewhat later, he came to an inn and decided to stay there. He saw a young woman sitting on the terrace, the daughter of the innkeeper. She was holding her cheek. Dr. Usui thought that she probably had a toothache and asked her: "May I help you?" The young woman was astonished but said: "Yes." Dr. Usui placed his hands on her cheek, and she felt better within just a few minutes. The young woman and her father were so happy about this that they invited Dr. Usui to a sumptuous meal. He thankfully accepted the invitation. Despite Dr. Usui's long period of fasting, the food agreed very well with him. The next afternoon, he continued on his way down into the valley. He soon reached the monastery, where his friend, the abbot, was already expecting him. The abbot was having considerable health problems at this time. He had an intense backache, but Dr. Usui was able to relieve his pain.

The next day, the two of them discussed what would be the best thing to do. They concluded that Dr. Usui should first take his newly acquired ability to a nearby impoverished neighborhood since the people there needed his help most urgently. During his first hours in the poor neighborhood, Dr. Usui walked through the streets with a burning torch in the light of day. When the people said to him: "Monk, what are you doing? It is still broad daylight," he responded: "I see only darkness here. If you want to learn something about the light, then come to me this evening."

Many people came, and he taught them the art of laying on hands. As a result, many people were healed. They were able to leave the poor neighborhood and find their way back into the society. Yet, after some time, Dr. Usui noticed that some of those who had already left the neighborhood were suddenly back again. When he asked them about this, they responded: "Everything is so difficult out there in the world. We feel better here. We don't have to do anything here." This caused Dr. Usui to ponder because he could not approve of such viewpoints. From this day on, it is said, he added two aspects to the teachings of Reiki: the five Reiki Principles as nourishment for the mind so that not only the diseases of the body but also the unhealthy attitudes would be healed and the maxim that anyone who wanted to learn Reiki from that time on had to also give something in exchange for it so they would value what they had received.

Dr. Usui continued his work, first in the poor neighborhood, and then in other places in Japan. As his life approached its end, he had initiated many people in Japan into Reiki. One of his close students, Dr. Hayashi, a physician and retired Marine officer, became his successor. After Usui's death, Dr. Hayashi opened a Reiki clinic in Tokyo. Using the background of his knowledge as a doctor, he began to record systematically the effects of Reiki.

One day, a young woman from Hawaii came to Dr. Hayashi's Reiki clinic. Her name was Hawayo Takata. She was a child of Japanese parents who had emigrated to Hawaii many years before. Hawayo Takata had come to Japan to have a difficult operation; she had a severe abdominal ailment, a tumor. When she was already on the

OP table, she had heard a voice that said to her: "The operation is not necessary." When she asked the physician whether there was a possibility for her other than the planned operation, Dr. Hayashi's Reiki clinic was recommended to her. Now she stood expectantly at the door of the clinic, and Dr. Hayashi welcomed her. In the time that followed, she received a daily treatment with Reiki until she was perfectly healed. As a result, Mrs. Takata was so enthusiastic about Reiki that she asked Dr. Hayashi to initiate her. However, Dr. Hayashi refused to do so because Mrs. Takata came from Hawaii and was not Japanese. Yet, Mrs. Takata did not give up. Instead, she got a letter of recommendation from a distinguished physician, the surgeon who initially had intended to do the planned operation for her, and returned to Dr. Hayashi with it. She finally succeeded in convincing Dr. Hayashi, and he initiated her into all three degrees of Reiki. Soon afterward, she went back to Hawaii and taught Reiki to the people there.

One night, Hawayo Takata had a dream about her teacher, Dr. Hayashi. The next morning, she intuitively knew that something important had happened and that her teacher needed her assistance. So she immediately left for Japan.

When she arrived at Dr. Hayashi's home and knocked on his door, he opened it for her and said: "I am happy that you have come, but it is still too early. Please spend some time with a colleague of mine who will teach you some things. I will let you know when the right time has come." Mrs. Takata did what was asked of her. When she received a telegram from Dr. Hayashi and returned to him a few weeks later, she discovered that the occasion for their meeting was a very sad one: It was in the period during the Second World War, shortly before Japan entered the combat. Since Dr. Hayashi was an officer of the Japanese navy, he feared that he would soon be drafted and forced to participate in the war. However, this would have gone against both his conscience and the consciousness that he had developed over the course of time. Consequently, he had decided to set a premature end to his life. He officially named Mrs. Takata as his successor, and within the scope of a solemn ceremony that was attended by only the closest relatives and students, he departed from this life.

In the period that followed, Mrs. Takata continued Dr. Hayashi's work on Hawaii and the American mainland. She dedicated the rest of her life to the teachings and practice of Reiki. Through her, Reiki came to the United States and spread to Europe from here. During the 1970s, after more than 30 years of experience with Reiki, Mrs. Takata began training a total of 22 Reiki Masters, including her granddaughter Phyllis Furumoto. Since the death of her grandmother in December of 1980, Phyllis Furumoto has been considered her successor.

Introduction

My Path with the History of the Usui System

Who was Mikao Usui really? What role did Dr. Hayashi play for the Usui System? How did Reiki come to the West? How did it continue to develop there? Is there something like the "true Reiki?" These and other questions crossed my mind in November of 2000 as I boarded the airplane that was to take me from Germany to the USA. I was on my way to Cataldo, Idaho, for my initiation into the Reiki Master Degree. I had already been initiated into the Usui System of Reiki for the past seven years. During the previous years, I had studied as a Master candidate with Paul David Mitchell, one of the 22 Masters who had originally been initiated by Hawayo Takata. Now the conclusion of my apprenticeship, the long-awaited initiation into the Master Degree, was about to take place.

Because the ten-hour flight meant a lot of sitting, I had some books with me including *The Spirit of Reiki,* which had just been published. The first section explores the history of the Usui System, together with new facts that had recently come to light. In recent years, people had begun to question the legendary form of the history of the Usui System as told by Mrs. Takata. After increasingly more new information about Mikao Usui, the founder of the Usui System, and his successor Dr. Hayashi, had reached the public, some of the details of the legendary history according to Hawayo Takata proved to be incorrect.

I leafed through the book, read one chapter or the other, and attempted to put together the pieces of the puzzle in my mind. So was the *Usui Reiki Ryoho Gakkai* actually the true successor organization of Mikao Usui? And was Dr. Hayashi just one of many who had continued the work of Usui? Nevertheless, Dr. Hayashi had done this with great success, as I discovered. And while the *Usui Reiki Ryoho Gakkai* had encapsulated itself from the outside world, Hawayo Takata, the successor of Dr. Hayashi, had brought the system into a form in which it ultimately spread around the world. And wasn't this the vision of Mikao Usui in keeping with everything that we know about him today: spreading Reiki throughout the world?

When I arrived at the airport in Spokane, Paul picked me up. I immediately felt the strong connection that we have. I know that this connection is always there, even when we don't see each other. But I always feel it time and again as a peak experience when we meet in person. We soon drove the car through the mountainous landscape, past the forests and lakes, finally arriving at the property of Paul and his family. It became dark quickly that evening, and I went to sleep early to overcome the time difference. Thoughts were simmering in my mind: Usui, Hayashi, Takata, myths, and legends. I am in Cataldo. The time has come. The truth—what is the truth?

The sun shone into my room the next morning. I got up and entered the kitchen, which is in the lower part of the *Dojo* where I was living with two other Master candidates. I made myself breakfast and Paul came over at some point. We drank coffee together.

During the following days, we had lessons during the day. In the evenings, the four of us often sat together and shared our thoughts and experiences with each other. Since I had become increasingly interested in the history of the Usui System, I asked many questions about it. I did this because many Masters I knew, including Paul, continued to tell the history in the legendary form according to Hawayo Takata, even though some of the information it contained had proved to be incorrect in the meantime. This was quite incomprehensible for me.

However, Paul taught us during these days in Cataldo that telling the story of the Reiki history is an obligatory component of a First Degree seminar. And since I was soon to also hold seminars myself and always took everything very seriously, I found myself in an inner conflict. I had an uneasy feeling about the legendary form of the Reiki history. Something within me rebelled, but something else said: "Stay calm! It's not that important. You can decide later."

The day of the initiation came, and it coincidentally fell on Thanksgiving. Phyllis Furumoto, who lived close by, had invited us to be her guests in the early evening. As we left the house to return home, we saw that it had started to snow. The first snow of the winter covered the landscape with its white dress. We drove back to the *Dojo* and decided that the moment for the initiation had come.

Some days later, I sat in the *Dojo* and thought about my future: What should I do when I returned to Germany? One thing was clear: I wanted to change my job! Why not take a risk and connect the two areas that were present in my life—journalism and Reiki—with each other? As I knew, Jürgen Kindler, the publisher of the German *Reiki Magazin,* had been searching for someone to run the magazine for the past several months. It was certain that I would not earn a great deal of money but I could leave my job as an employee behind me and venture into a new field. Yes, I decided to ask Jürgen!

The last days in the *Dojo* were very peaceful. I was completely alone—the two women had already left for the airport—and sometimes Paul came over or I visited him. I took little walks and explored the Idaho countryside.

Back in Berlin, I called Jürgen and arranged a meeting. It was before Christmas, and the streets and houses were decorated with colorful lights. I walked through the evening darkness, as if drawn by invisible strings, into my future. Jürgen and I very quickly agreed on the terms. I gave notice at my old job and began working for the German-language *Reiki Magazin.*

After an initial, difficult phase of orientation, during which I had to become acquainted with the new circumstances, I felt that I was completely in my element. From the very beginning, I was especially concerned with making a contribution through the magazine to create a better information situation regarding the history of the Usui System. I took stock of it in a longer article, and then we started a new series on this topic.

In my Reiki seminars, I attempted to tell the history in its legendary form. However, I often thought: "Everyone must notice that it isn't entirely correct." So this sometimes resulted in critical questions coming from the seminar participants. Soon I began to make some changes to the beginning, taking out information that I perceived to be incorrect. Yet, this somehow did not appear to be right in terms of the energy. The question was: Was there a problem with the changes themselves or that I was not really happy with making the changes? I do not know. And, in all honesty: In retrospect I cannot say whether the history profited in any way through my changes. Furthermore, as an irony of fate, I soon had to take some of the changes out again because it turned out that they were also based on incorrect information. This was the moment in which I capitulated. I began once again to tell the history in its old form. Then, for the first time, I found my way to its inner essence.

In the meantime, I have decided upon the following approach to the history: Before I tell it in its old, legendary form in seminars, I point out that this is a type of legend. In addition, I speak of Mikao Usui not as a "Christian priest" but as a "scholar," as Paul, my Reiki Teacher, once formulated it in a seminar that I attended as a guest. Moreover, I mention that Mikao Usui studied both Buddhist and Christian scriptures during his search since this has been confirmed by the inscription on his memorial stone at the Saihoji Temple in Tokyo.

With time I have discovered that recounting the history does not primarily involve imparting information. Instead, its main purpose is to make sure that the seminar participants attain a feeling for the nature of Reiki. In its legendary form, the history carries a certain energy that is valuable for Reiki students in making contact with the universal life energy. This is why the Reiki history is told within the scope of a First Degree seminar. In my experience, no one in a First Degree seminar is actually interested in detailed information about the history of the Usui System. And those who want to know more later on will find the appropriate information in books like this.

For myself, I can say the following: Now that I have found my way back to the legendary form of the history, I can also write a book about everything that this history leaves out. Without finding my way back to it, I would probably have only taken a stance against the old form of the history and used the pages of the book for a personal confrontation with the Reiki tradition from which I come. Now that I have made my peace with the old form, I can let go of it again and write this book. And when this book is done, I will be open to whatever comes next.

1. The Beginnings
Mikao Usui and Reiki Ryoho

Very little is known about the life and work of Mikao Usui. Although there are many references and assumptions about his path in life from a great variety of sources, it is still not clear what the truth is and what is just a legend. One of the few reliable sources is the inscription on the memorial stone at the Saihoji Temple in Tokyo.[1] The memorial stone was erected in February of 1927, about one year after Mikao Usui's death, by some of his students in the sincere memory of him and his work. The inscription is written in the old Japanese characters, which even makes them difficult for modern Japanese to understand. For people of the West, a complicating factor is that translations from Japanese always bring inaccuracies with them since the Japanese language is full of ambiguity.

The Life Path of Mikao Usui

According to the inscription on the memorial stone, Mikao Usui was born on August 15, 1865 in Japan. Furthermore, it says: "Even during his childhood he learned diligently, even under difficult conditions, so that his abilities were far superior to his peers. When he became an adult, he went to Europe and America and studied in China. But his career did not progress, as he would have liked it to. He was not lucky, and was often in financial need. Despite everything, he did not give up one bit but worked on himself even more diligently than before."[2]

In terms of the circumstances that led to the development of the Reiki method of healing by Mikao Usui, the inscription of the memorial stone does not provide any clear information. This could be because the students of Usui who erected the memorial stone may not have known much about it themselves or believed that this type of information did not belong on a memorial stone accessible to the public. Another aspect is that they did not even write the inscription themselves but apparently had it done by a professional obituary writer.[3]

About one year after my initiation into the Master Degree, I began to be quite interested in the life and work of Mikao Usui. I had already held my first Reiki seminars, in the tradition of *Usui Shiki Ryoho,* as I had learned it from my teacher, Paul Mitchell. This system of Reiki has primarily been shaped by Dr. Hayashi, one of the successors of Mikao Usui, as well as by Hawayo Takata, the successor of Dr. Hayashi. This is how the Reiki method of healing developed into the form in which it has ultimately spread around the world. *Usui Shiki Ryoho* means the "Usui System of Natural Healing." After an initial phase of internalizing this system and transmitting the first two degrees of this system to others, I was now open for integrating new impulses into my own Reiki path.

During an interview that I had with the English Reiki Teacher Don Alexander about the origins of Reiki, I felt very touched by the way he spoke and by what he said. Don discovered the Usui System of Reiki for himself in 1985. Soon after that, he also began to teach it. Since then he has dedicated his life to, as he calls it, "researching the living correlations" from where Mikao Usui's teachings came. He is a practicing Buddhist and, before he began his path with Reiki, spent many years living as a monk in a Buddhist monastery in Thailand. For Don, the Usui System of Reiki is primarily a spiritual path; this is a perspective that he has derived directly from Mikao Usui.

Meditation Practice

At a symbol seminar with Don in which I participated, I received an abundance of information and stories about the Reiki symbols.

As sources for his knowledge, Don named his teachers Chris Marsh and Andy Bowling, as well as an early student of Mikao Usui, a Buddhist nun by the name of Suzuki-San, who is now said to be more than one-hundred years old. In addition to the extensive knowledge about the Reiki symbols in his seminars, Don teaches various techniques that date back to Mikao Usui, including the exercise of *Hatsureiho*. This is a meditation practice that Mikao Usui taught primarily to those students who felt the desire to progress further in their practice. *Hatsu* means something like "start" or "stimulate," *rei* is the "rei" of Reiki, and ho means method.[4] As confirmed by various sources, Mikao Usui apparently recommended that his students do this exercise, which is illustrated on pages 22–24 as instructed by Don Alexander.

The Principles

Another important element of Usui's teachings were the Reiki Principles. Mikao Usui reportedly encouraged his students to recite the Principles every morning and every evening and translate them into reality in their everyday lives. This was apparently even the heart of practicing the Reiki method of healing at that time, according to the inscription of the memorial stone for Mikao Usui. It says: "The heart of learning this method is reciting the Five Principles mornings and evenings while meditatively sitting still in the *Gassho* posture and repeating them mentally, which cultivates a pure and healthy mind, and turning the five Principles into reality in everyday life."[5]

A translation of the original version of the five Principles is:

> Just for today,
>
> Don't get angry.
> Don't worry.
> Be grateful.
> Work hard.
> Be kind to others.[6]

Hatsureiho Meditation
According to Mikao Usui, as instructed by Don Alexander

The exercise will help you strengthen your practice of Reiki and will support your spiritual path.

1. Posture

Sit in Seiza (kneeling Japanese style), cross-legged (yogi style), or, if preferred, on an upright chair. If about to offer a treatment session, you might prefer to stand.

Sit comfortably and become aware of your body. Feel the shape and the weight of your body. Your consciousness is in your body and not in your mind. Feel deeply as though you were asking yourself—and feeling for the answer: "How are my bones feeling just now?" Allow your breath to come and go naturally, just as your body's wisdom chooses for it to be.

2. Gassho

Put your hands together in a respectful salutation … and feel how your consciousness changes as you move into this gesture. Notice what happens to your consciousness as you do this.

3. Mokunen: Concentration and clear intention

Having felt this gesture of Gassho, hold the very clear intention: "Now I begin Hatsureiho!"

4. Kenyoku: Dry bathing or brushing off to clear the energy field

Put your right hand on your left shoulder and brush downwards diagonally across the body to your right hip. If it is more comfortable, you may brush downwards within the energy field a few centimeters from the body.

Do the same thing with your left hand: Put it on the right shoulder and brush downward diagonally across the body to your left hip. Repeat the brush with your right hand: Stretch your left arm forward slightly, palms facing up. Now with the fingers of your right hand to the palm of your left, and the thumb of your right hand sandwiching from the back of the left, brush vigorously from wrist to beyond your left fingertips. Repeat on the other side. And again on the left.

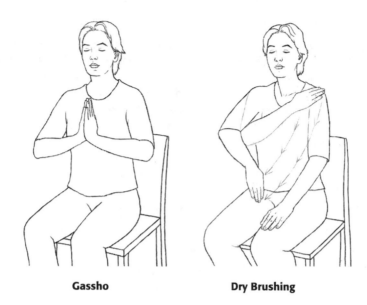

Gassho   **Dry Brushing**

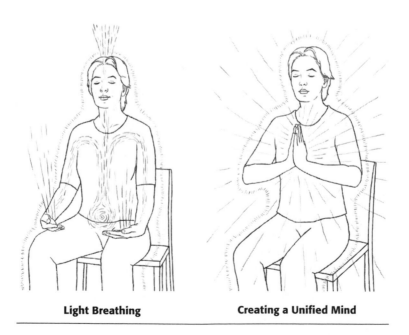

Light Breathing   **Creating a Unified Mind**

5. Joshin Kokyu ho: Focusing the mind on one thing with breath

As you now hold your hands, palms upward, you can visualize the pure light of Reiki flowing into your body through your crown chakra ... and through your hands ... and down to the Hara*. So you have these three streams of light coming into your body with each in-breath. And with each out-breath, visualize that this light in the Hara gets brighter and expands throughout all of the pores of your skin ... to illuminate and heal the space ... and everyone all around. And you continue breathing like this ... bringing the light in ... and out ... expanding the light to heal all around ... for a count of at least 10 breaths ... longer if you wish. It is wonderful if you want to practice in this way for a thousand breaths, but it shouldn't be any less than 10.

(*Hara is a Japanese term that refers to a center of energy and gravity in our body located just below the navel.)

So now you are sitting here as a being of light, breathing light in and breathing light out ... the light of enlightenment, the light of healing, the light of Reiki ... and all the while you are feeling your body and feeling the Hara ... As you practice, allow yourself to smile. This is a happy practice.

6. Gassho

Put your hands together in a respectful salutation.

7. Seishin Toitsu: Creating a unified mind

And as you inhale, visualize that this great light of Reiki is coming in through the hands and streaming down into the Hara ... As you breathe out, filling the body as before, stream the light out through your gassho-joined hands ... to illumine and heal the space ... and everyone all around. Again, practice in this way for an absolute minimum of 10 breaths.

8. Mokunen: Focus with clear intention

And when you know that it is time to close, have the clear intention: "Now I finish, now I end, now I complete this practice of Hatsureiho!" (Use whichever term gives you a precise feeling of completion.) And as you have that clear intention, put your hands down ... and open your eyes.

The original version in Japanese is:

Kyo dake wa
Ikaru-na
Shinpai suna
Kansha shite
Gyo hage me
Hito ni shinsetsu ni[7]

The contents of the Principles did not come from Mikao Usui alone. Instead, they originated in the broad field of Japanese or Asian philosophy. As Hiroko Kasahara explained to me during our work on her translation of the memorial-stone inscription, every Japanese person is familiar with the essential aspects of this philosophy, even without knowing about Reiki. Similar contents are also found in the wisdom teachings of Confucius. The Principles may also to date back to a book with the title *Kenzen no Genri* (English: The Principle of Health) by Dr. Bizan Suzuki, which was published in 1914 in Japan. A portion of it reads: "Just for today, don't get angry, don't be afraid, be honest, work hard, and be kind to others."

As the memorial-stone inscription says, Mikao Usui spoke of the Principles as "the secret method of achieving happiness." He also called them "the miracle cure against all diseases."[8]

Reiju Energy Transmission

In his seminars and at the regular meetings with his students, it is reported that Mikao Usui gave *Reiju* energy transmissions. According to Hiroko Kasahara, this was the original form of the initiation. *Rei* is the *Rei* of Reiki and *ju* means "transmission from teacher to student." However, it appears that Usui never spoke about an "initiation" but more of a "transmission of the *Rei.*" In learning the First Degree, which in Japanese is called *Shoden* (which means something like "fundamental teaching"), just one initiation, that is a "transmission of Rei," was given at that time. But Mikao Usui always made it very clear that it was especially important to participate in the regular meetings, in which there were additional *Reiju* energy transmissions to constantly increase the flow of the universal energy within oneself.[9] As a source for her knowledge, Hiroko Kasahara cited her teacher Hiroshi Doi (cf. pg. 165).

Reiki Ryoho

As previously mentioned, we know very little about the context from which Mikao Usui created the Reiki method of healing. The inscription on the memorial stone contains the expression *Reiki Ryoho* as the name for the practice that he developed. Here, *Reiki* means "the universal life energy," Ryo means something like "heal," and ho means "method." So the literal translation of the name *Reiki Ryoho* represents something like the "Reiki Healing Method."

In one place of the memorial-stone inscription, we learn more about the person of Mikao Usui, as well as the areas of knowledge in which he was proficient: "Usui Sensei had a gentle and modest nature and placed little value on superficial things. He had a strong stature and always showed a friendly smile. But when it was important, he proved to have a strong will. He was very patient and prudent. He was talented in many ways and well-read in every sense. For example, he was familiar with the areas of history, biography, medical books, the religious scriptures of Buddhism and Christianity, the area of psychology, the art of *Shinsen,* as well as the areas of incantation, oracles, and physiognomics."[10]

Usui Sensei

Seen in this light, Mikao Usui was also a very experienced man. He had traveled the world, including Europe, America, and China, and had acquired many different types of knowledge. In another part of the memorial-stone inscription, it becomes clear that he was shown great respect by everyone. In Japanese there is an expression that people can use when they want to demonstrate their respect for someone: *Sensei.* For example, this word can be added after a person's name when someone speaks or writes about him. For this reason, the expression *Usui Sensei* for Mikao Usui is customary among Japanese Reiki practitioners.

As far as I know, the phrase "Dr. Usui" is rarely used in Japan. The memorial-stone inscription does not mention that Mikao Usui had a doctorate. Even if it appears that he was familiar with medical writings, he was certainly not a physician because we can assume that this would have been mentioned in an obituary. So why is it that Reiki practitioners in the West generally speak of "Dr. Usui"? As far as I know, the term "Dr. Usui" goes back to Dr. Hayashi. As Paul Mitchell mentioned in an interview that I had with him in October of 2003, a certificate signed by a notary that was prepared by Dr. Hayashi for his successor Hawayo Takata had various translations into English for the name of the practice that he was transmitting to her. One of them is: "Dr. Usui's Reiki System of Healing."[11]

Why is he referred to as "Dr. Usui" here? We don't know. Was it because Dr. Hayashi, who himself had a genuine title of doctor (he was a navy physician), did not want to place himself above his esteemed teacher? Or was it because, as a medical professional, Dr. Hayashi thought there would be a greater social acceptance of the term "Dr. Usui's Reiki System of Healing"? Or is the use of the title of doctor for Mikao Usui simply an attempt to translate the Japanese *Sensei* into English? The expression *Sensei* is used in Japanese not only in a personal context but also in a very general way: For example, *Sensei* is a term bestowed upon all teachers, professors, physicians, delegates, attorneys, and authors. A further possibility is that Mikao Usui actually had a doctorate but it was an honorary doctorate, according to an (unfortunately) unverified source on the Internet. But why isn't anything written about this in the memorial-stone inscription?

Be that as it may: I have decided not to use "Dr. Usui" or "Usui Sensei" in this book but simply speak of Mikao Usui. This is my way of honoring his person in view of the impenetrable abundance of claims that are currently circulating about him. Incidentally, I was surprised to discover while working with Hiroko Kasahara on her translation of the memorial-stone inscription that Mikao Usui also had a type of pen name, something that was not unusual in the Japan of that era for a scholar. Mikao Usui's pen name, or we could even call it his poetic name, was: *Gyohan*. This means something like: "the sail in the light of dawn."[12]

Mount Kurama

There are many legends about Mikao Usui's experience on Mount Kurama near Kyoto. Mount Kurama is considered to be a special sacred place. Numerous temples of various spiritual traditions are located there, and the mountain is called the "spiritual heart of Japan." It is said that Mikao Usui was given the knowledge of Reiki on Mount Kurama while in deep meditation. Some say that he attained enlightenment as a result. Others are more reserved in stating that he had an experience of enlightenment. The memorial-stone inscription makes this comment: "One day he climbed up Mount Kurama. He fasted there and practiced intensely for 21 days. On the 21st day, he felt the great Reiki energy above his head and felt himself opened and completely free of any doubt. He received *Reiki Ryoho.*"[13]

In the following period, he tried out the newly acquired ability on himself and his family, which included his wife Sadako, his son Fuji, and his daughter.[14] Within the shortest amount of time, the positive effects were obvious. As a result, he decided not to keep this ability just for himself alone but pass it on to people everywhere. In April of 1922, he began to work as a teacher and healer in Tokyo. Furthermore, the memorial-stone inscription says: "He transmitted *Reiki Ryoho* and carried out treatments. The area in front of his door was full of the shoes from people who came from near and far to his classes or treatments."[15]

The Big Earthquake

About one-and-a-half years after Usui had gone to Tokyo, there was a major earthquake in which most of the city burned down. This earthquake was especially disastrous, which is why it is still remembered generally in all of Japan, even today. The memorial-stone inscription comments that: "The suffering groans of the many injured and sick could be heard everywhere. This deeply hurt Usui Sensei, and he walked through the city day after day. No one knows how many people were saved by his treatment. In any case, Usui Sensei rescued many who were suffering due to this plight."[16]

As we know, there is no mention of an earthquake anywhere in the legendary form of the history, as told by Hawayo Takata. Instead, Mrs. Takata told us that Mikao Usui spent some time in a poor quarter after his experience on Mount Kurama. Since there is in turn no mention of Usui's work in an impoverished neighborhood in the memorial-stone inscription, we can assume here that the help Usui gave to the needy after the earthquake was merged in the legend with an episode in which Usui took care of those in need in an impoverished area. This may have occurred with the goal of packing some essential teachings into the history.

The Degrees of Reiki Ryoho

After the big earthquake, people everywhere in Tokyo hurried to quickly rebuild the city. With time, more and more individuals came to Mikao Usui. About one-and-a-half years after the earthquake, the house in which he lived in Tokyo became too small for the substantial rush of people. So he moved into a larger house that was built in a suburb of Tokyo, in Nakano.[17]

Anyone who wanted to learn the Reiki method of healing at that time was offered, as Hiroko Kasahara describes it[18], a system of three degrees and six ranks. While the degree structure was related to learning the Reiki method, the rank order was related to the individual abilities as a Reiki practitioner. The First Degree was called *Shoden,* which means something like "fundamental teaching." This First Degree was related to the lower four ranks. Anyone participating in a seminar of the First Degree was automatically classified in the lowest rank, the Sixth Rank. In order to reach the additional three ranks that were connected with the First Degree, special abilities were required as a Reiki practitioner. These focused on the development of one's intuition and the ability to be a pure channel (cf. pg. 46). People were only allowed to register for the Second Degree when they had adequately developed these abilities. When this had been successfully accomplished, a person was then elevated to the Third Rank. With the attainment of the Third Rank, it was finally possible to reach the Second Degree.

The Second Degree was called *Okuden,* which means something like "the deepest or last teaching." This degree was intended to be taught in two separate instructional units, according to Tadao Yamaguchi[19]: in *Okuden-Zenki* and *Okuden-Koki.* The technique of distant healing was said to only be conveyed in the second part. However, the Second Degree was apparently offered in a complete form as a course for students who had traveled great distances.

Furthermore, there was the Third Degree, *Shinpiden*, which only a few people attained during the lifetime of Usui. *Shinpiden* means something like "teaching of the mystery." Mikao Usui allowed only those who had achieved a certain degree of personal and spiritual maturity and whose consciousness he considered highly developed to participate in this degree. It was not possible to reach any other levels of rank beyond the Third Rank, no matter what degree a person had. This is because Mikao Usui had placed himself in the Second Rank.[20]

The Poems of the Meiji Emperor

At Usui's regular meetings with his students, in addition to the Reiju energy transmissions and the recitation of the Principles, there was probably a third component that he saw as especially valuable: the poetry of the Meiji Emperor. The Meiji Emperor was an emperor in Japan who was loved by all. He ruled the country for an unusually long period of 45 years with great success. The emperors are not called by their personal names in Japan but by the names of the periods during which they ruled. The Meiji Emperor's personal name was Mutsuhito. *Meiji* means something like "enlightened government." This term characterizes the nature of the period of this emperor's regency, under which a general enlightenment and opening occurred in the country. The Meiji Emperor came into office in 1868. Mikao Usui was born three years earlier. The Meiji Emperor governed the country in the time from 1868-1912, which is during the largest portion of Mikao Usui's lifetime.

The Meiji Emperor was very popular with the Japanese people. He reportedly wrote more than 100,000 poems during his lifetime. Mikao Usui felt high esteem for the Meiji Emperor and selected 125 of his poems for spiritual purposes. These played an important role in his instruction and at the regular meetings with his students. They all recited some of these poems together at the beginning of each meeting. Moreover, Mikao Usui recommended that his students learn the poetry as food for the spirit.[21] Here is one of these poems in translation:

> The Spirit
>
> Whatever happens
> In any situation
> It is my wish that
> The spirit remains
> Without boundaries (free)[22]

In those days, in which affirmation techniques had not yet been developed, this poetry may have also served as affirmations, as Hiroko Kasahara ascertains in her German-language article on Reiki in Japan, which appeared in the *Reiki Magazin*.[23]

Death in Fukuyama

Once Mikao Usui's work became well-known, he was invited by many people to various areas of Japan. As a result, one day he left on a longer journey from which he would not return: He went to Kure and Hiroshima, traveled on to Saga, and then finally went to Fukuyama. He unexpectedly became ill there and died in an inn.[24] This was on March 9, 1926. Mikao Usui was 61 years of age.

He may have had the following poem by the Meiji Emperor on his mind during his last hours:

> People
>
> Things may not seem to work out
> As you wish
> But they turn out to be good
> When you look back
> At your (own) life[25]

Various Historical Sources

As we have already established, there are various sources that differ in part in their statements about the life and work of Mikao Usui. Two main currents can be recognized at this time: One includes information that came from the members of the *Usui Reiki Ryoho Gakkai,* one of Mikao Usui's successor organizations (see pg. 37). The essential points of this information are presented on the last pages. Furthermore, there is a current of partially differing information, which is primarily based on the knowledge of the English Reiki Teacher Chris Marsh. Chris Marsh is apparently in contact with an early student of Mikao Usui, Suzuki-San who was born in 1895 and, it was said, was already one of his students in 1915. She is reportedly still alive today. Don Alexander, who based large portions of his seminar contents on it, also makes use of this knowledge. According to this source, the Reiki method was not primarily a method of healing for Mikao Usui. Instead, the spiritual aspect was always in the foreground. And, above all, this was influenced by Buddhism and not Taoism, which may be the impression created by the memorial-stone inscription's statement that Usui undertook a journey to study in China and had good knowledge in the area of *Shinsen.*

In the words of Don Alexander, he experiences Mikao Usui as someone who was a spiritually highly evolved Buddhist practitioner and followed Tendai Buddhism. The family from which Usui came was reportedly an old Samurai clan; as a result, Usui also learned and practiced the martial arts, among other things. In terms of the practice of *Reiki Ryoho,* Usui initially used various meditation techniques and taught the so-called *Kotodamas.* These are "sacred sounds" that are chanted like mantras (cf. pg. 220). On the other hand, the symbols were not even part of the practice at the beginning. They were only added later to facilitate the access to the practice. The first statement would fit in well with the comments in

33

the memorial-stone inscription that Mikao Usui was well-versed in the area of incantation (cf. pg. 26). For the latter statement, there are currently no confirmations or contradictory information to be found in other sources.

Another unclear area relates to the dates for Mikao Usui's experiences on Mount Kurama. The general assumption is that this occurred in the year 1922. However, the inscription of the memorial stone does not clarify this point. Another question is whether Mikao Usui's experience on Mount Kurama, as described by the memorial-stone inscription and the legendary form of the history according to Hawayo Takata, actually had the outstanding significance for the development of the Reiki method. Based on the information from Chris Marsh, Mikao Usui had already discovered a many decisive aspects of the Reiki method some years before 1922 and had previously begun to teach them.

However, if we look at the careers of spiritual personalities, we discover that they usually had many different phases in their lives. Perhaps the unclear aspects in terms of Mikao Usui's work simply are related to the fact that some of the sources refer to early phases in his life (about which the memorial-stone inscription reveals very little) and other sources point to the later phase of his work.

I believe what ultimately counts are the experiences we have today with the teachers we are in contact with and from whom we learn. And this also includes the teachers whose seminars we attend to learn more about the teachings of Mikao Usui. For example, I was able to learn a great deal from Don Alexander, quite apart from whether or not he told me something about Mikao Usui.

The Truth About Mikao Usui?

Within the scope of my research for this book, this much has become clear to me: There cannot be "one" truth about Mikao Usui. Like other figures of world history, new correlations relating to the person of Mikao Usui become known repeatedly in the course of time, permitting fresh insights into his life and work. At the same time, we must continue to ask what the truth actually is, what is an interpretation of it, and what are just assumptions. Even if many of the Reiki practitioners would like to have it this way: Something like "the teachings of Mikao Usui," to which we can simply and easily refer, apparently do not exist. Or at least today, it appears that almost all of the doors that lead to this are closed to a large extent. This is a situation that we can only accept as Reiki practitioners. And perhaps this insight can help, after a phase of natural interest in the formation period of the Usui System, to once again concentrate on our own practice.

⌣⟶

Mikao Usui is frequently called the founder of the Usui System of Reiki. However, a founder usually has a high degree of lasting, form-giving influence on the system that he or she has established. For example, this is the case with the system of the Bach Flowers, founded by Dr. Edward Bach (see pg. 184), as well as for the Aura-Soma system, which goes back to Vicky Wall (see pg. 191). Both systems, similar to the Usui System, make existing energies popular and available to a greater amount of people in a special way. In terms of the Bach Flowers and the Aura-Soma system, the form-giving influence of their founders still fundamentally determines them today, although many years have passed since their death. However, the form-giving influence of Mikao Usui on the modern expressions of the system is now barely perceptible in the Usui System of Reiki.

In view of the immense variety of forms in the current worldwide Reiki scene, the question arises whether the term "founder" actually still describes the person of Mikao Usui.

Here is a comparison: In the area of religious studies, the term "founder of a religion" has now often been replaced by "establisher of a religion." The modern perspective is that the teachings and work of a founding figure are not identical with the religion that is connected with him. When I look at the current situation in terms of Reiki, I discover that this thought is also appropriate for the "world of Reiki." Hardly any of the forms of the Usui System of Reiki practiced by millions of people throughout the world is still identical with what Mikao Usui taught in his day. So it would perhaps be better to see him as an "establishing figure" rather than as the founder of the Usui System of Reiki. Someone who establishes something makes a gift of it, passes it on, and simultaneously detaches himself somewhat from it. In contrast to the work of a founder, the work of an establisher is less specific. It tends to be more setting something in motion or preparing the soil so that it can develop.

It is my feeling that we can best do justice to the work of Mikao Usui—and therefore also to his person—if we keep him in our mind and hearts in this way: as the establisher of the Usui System of Reiki, as a pioneer in the application of the universal life energy on earth.

2. Continuation

The Students of Mikao Usui

Up to the time of his death, Mikao Usui had initiated about 2,000 people into Reiki.[1] However, there were only a handful of students who he initiated into the Third Degree *(Shinpiden)*. This group reportedly included about 20 people, three of which were women.[2] According to the research by Frank Arjava Petter and Dave King, the following seven people were part of this circle: Juzaburo Ushida, Dr. Chujiro Hayashi, Toshihiro Eguchi, Toyoichi Wanami, Ilichi Taketomi, Kozo Ogawa, and Yoshiharu Watanabe.[3]

The Usui Reiki Ryoho Gakkai

After Mikao Usui's death, the larger community that had formed during his lifetime was dissolved to a great extent. What remained was the *Usui Reiki Ryoho Gakkai* that, according to the inscription of the memorial stone, had been established by Usui himself during his lifetime. After Usui's death, one of the students who he had initiated into the Third Degree *(Shinpiden)*—Juzaburo Ushida—became the President of the *Usui Reiki Ryoho Gakkai*. Many of Usui's students took their own paths after that time.[4] In the following period, very few of them remained members of the *Usui Reiki Ryoho Gakkai*. *Gakkai* means something like "society." So *Usui Reiki Ryoho Gakkai* can be approximately translated to mean "the society of the Reiki method of healing according to Usui."

A great service by the *Usui Reiki Ryoho Gakkai* is that it has preserved and cultivated the legacy of the *Reiki Ryoho* according to Mikao Usui up into the present day. It has an uninterrupted series of presidents who each headed the society during a certain time period. According to the research by William Lee Rand, these were the presidents of the *Usui Reiki Ryoho Gakkai*[5] up to now. The following list begins with Juzaburo Ushida, the first president after Usui's death:

Mr. Juzaburo Ushida
Mr. Kanichi Taketomi
Mr. Yoshiharu Watanabe
Mr. Hoichi Wanami
Ms. Kimiko Koyama
Mr. Masayoshi Kondo

The fact that the *Usui Reiki Ryoho Gakkai* has preserved a handbook that Mikao Usui put together for his students and that this handbook has now reached the public makes it possible for us to get an impression of what Mikao Usui found valuable enough to write down. The handbook includes various sections:

- A formal explanation by Usui of why he teaches Reiki to the public
- Various questions to Usui regarding *Reiki Ryoho* and Usui's responses to them
- A "treatment plan," which is an overview of the standard hand positions for the treatment of specific body parts and diseases
- The 125 poems of the Meiji Emperor, which Usui had selected for the spiritual work

(For more about the contents of this handbook, see Chapter 6, starting on pg. 149)

As Mikao Usui expressed in his explanation of why he teaches Reiki in public, he placed much importance on spreading the Reiki method of healing in a major way. The inscription on the memorial stone contains passages that are in a similar vein. They say that the successful spreading of *Reiki Ryoho* would "make a large contribution toward saving the earth and expanding the consciousness of the people. (…) Usui *Sensei* is dead, but *Reiki Ryoho* must continue to spread for a long time to come and throughout the world. That Usui Sensei passed on to the people what he had acquired himself was truly a great deed!"[6]

In Usui's explanation of why he teaches Reiki to the public, he said: "Our *Reiki Ryoho* is something absolutely original and cannot be compared with any other (spiritual) path in the world. This is why I would like to make this method (freely) available to the public for the well-being of humanity. Each of us has the potential of being given a gift by the divine, which results in the body and soul becoming unified. In this way (with Reiki), a great many people will experience the blessing of the divine."[7]

With this explanation, Usui strongly differentiated his plans of teaching Reiki to the public from the traditional approach of "keeping a found secret for oneself." In the explanation of this, he said: "From time immemorial, it has often happened that someone who has found an original, secret law has either kept it for himself or only shared it with his descendents. This secret was then used as security in life for his descendents. (...) The secret is not passed on to outsiders. However, this is an old-fashioned custom from the last century (and therefore outdated)."[8]

Yet, the Usui's express wish to have the Reiki method of healing spread widely did not occur through the *Usui Reiki Ryoho Gakkai*. Instead, through the years it increasingly became a type of secret society. There were also historical reasons for this development. The location of the headquarters of the *Usui Reiki Ryoho Gakkai*, as described by Hiroko Kasahara, had to be moved a number of times during the Second World War because of the many bombardments. The main path upon which the Reiki method of healing had been spread at this time was within the Japanese navy. So Juzaburo Ushida, the President of the *Usui Reiki Ryoho Gakkai*, as well as his successor, Kanichi Taketomi, and also another successor,

Hoichi Wanami, were all admirals of the Japanese navy. In the memorial-stone inscription, "cities such as Kure, Hiroshima, Saga, and Fukuyama were mentioned, which Usui Sensei had visited upon invitation. There were navy harbors in all of these cities. After the war, this basis for spreading Reiki was destroyed, as well as the Japanese navy itself.

After the war, Kimiko Koyama took over the *Usui Reiki Ryoho Gakkai.* But now even less people in Japan were interested in a method of healing like Reiki. After the Japanese had lost the war, they had to thoroughly obliterate, virtually wipe out, everything that they had believed in before, such as the myth surrounding the emperor family. They experienced an unimaginable upheaval of their concepts of values. Japanese society became increasingly oriented toward material values. The number of members in the *Usui Reiki Ryoho Gakkai* decreased dramatically, and it had to survive several severe crises."[9]

Since the change in values in Japan after the Second World War caused a transformation in the population's thinking regarding the traditional methods of healing, it is plausible that the *Usui Reiki Ryoho Gakkai* did not continue to spread the Reiki healing method during this phase. But what is surprising is that this society totally avoids communication with the public to this day, especially shunning contact with foreigners. For example, Frank Arjava Petter reports the following episode in his book *Reiki Fire:* After he had received the telephone number of the *Usui Reiki Ryoho Gakkai* from one of his students, he called it within the scope of researching his book: "The person who answered the phone asked us not to publish her name. She said that she did not intend to read my book and did not want to have anything to do with Reiki 'that comes from outside of Japan'! She also mentioned that she had been approached by a Japanese individual who teaches Reiki in New York, but had refused to meet that person."[10]

Other people have also reported similar experiences when attempting to establish contact with the *Usui Reiki Ryoho Gakkai*. Be that as it may, the worldwide spreading of the Reiki healing method, as we know, was not destined to occur through the *Usui Reiki Ryoho Gakkai* but took a completely different course: namely through Dr. Hayashi and Hawayo Takata.

Dr. Chujiro Hayashi

Dr. Hayashi was apparently first a member of the *Usui Reiki Ryoho Gakkai*. However, he soon left this society and carried on the Reiki method of healing that Usui had taught him in his own way. He founded his own society, the *Hayashi Reiki Kenkyukai* (Hayashi Reiki Research Society) and actively promoted the dissemination of Reiki throughout all of Japan.[11]

Dr. Hayashi was born on September 15, 1880 in Tokyo. Like Mikao Usui, he was married and had two children, a son and a daughter. And like some of the presidents of the *Usui Reiki Ryoho Gakkai*, he also belonged to the Japanese navy. He did not have the rank of an admiral like the early presidents of the *Usui Reiki Ryoho Gakkai*, but that of a colonel; this rank is directly beneath that of an admiral in the hierarchy.[12] In the year 1918, he was the commander of the defense station of Port Ominato. Kanichi Taketomi, Juzaburo Ushida's successor in the *Usui Reiki Ryoho Gakkai*, was the chief of staff here.[13]

Together with the founding of the *Hayashi Reiki Kenkyukai* during the mid-1920s, Dr. Hayashi established a Reiki clinic in Tokyo. According to information from Chiyoko Yamaguchi, one of Dr. Hayashi's students, there were a total of ten tables upon which the patients were treated by two practitioners each.[14] Dr. Hayashi probably also placed special emphasis on the treatment of the meridians, reflexology points, and energy centers. Through his experiences as a physician, he apparently felt that he was capable of creating his own index of hand positions, which he summarized in a new overview, the *Ryoho Shishin* (Treatment Plan for the Healing Method).[15] However, this differed in very few points from the treatment plan according to Mikao Usui. Both treatment plans consist of a detailed list of various hand positions for the treatment of diseases and physical problems (cf. pgs. 156 ff.). Dr. Hayashi imparted his treatment plan, as well as the poetry of the Meiji Emperor (see pg. 31) to his students, together with fans in the Japanese style upon which the Reiki Principles were written.[16]

In both Tokyo and Osaka, Dr. Hayashi held a monthly seminar in *Shoden,* the First Degree. He also traveled to other cities in Japan, holding seminars there at larger intervals. A *Shoden* seminar usually lasted four or five days. There were *Reiju* energy transmissions in the mornings, then instruction, and in the afternoons the practitioners practiced and gave each other sessions. Dr. Hayashi kept the system of the three degrees and six ranks according to Mikao Usui. During a *Shoden* seminar, he often also imparted the contents of all the related ranks (the ranks from 5 to 3, cf. pg. 30) in addition to the usual material. It generally took a few months, sometimes even up to a year or longer, until the participants had developed their intuition and abilities as treatment-givers to the point that they could fulfill the requirements of these ranks (cf. pg. 46). Anyone who had reached the Third Rank could subsequently learn *Okuden,* the Second Degree.[17]

In terms of the Third Degree, *Shinpiden,* according to Tadao Yamaguchi[18], at the time of Dr. Hayashi there was a subdivision of this degree into *Shihan* (teacher) and *Shihan Kaku* (teacher's assistant). A *Shihan Kaku* was already empowered to give the *Reiju* energy transmissions. This made it possible for ongoing meetings of his students, which included *Reiju* energy transmissions, to be held even in places to which Dr. Hayashi traveled just rarely as soon as someone there had reached this preliminary stage to the Third Degree. (We currently do not know whether such a subdivision of the Third Degree into two levels had also been customary during the time of Mikao Usui; at least there is nothing to this effect in the currently available sources.) In addition to Tokyo, which was the location of the Reiki clinic and the *Hayashi Reiki Kenkyukai,* Dr. Hayashi had branches in many other Japanese cities. He and his wife frequently traveled there to hold seminars. For example, there were branches in Osaka, Daishiji, and Ishiwaka.[19]

Recognition Effect

When I read the book *The Hayashi Reiki Manual*[20] in the summer of 2003, I felt very connected with the contents of this book in some parts. Thanks to the research of Frank Arjava Petter, a book was available for the first time to provide information about the life and work of Dr. Hayashi. In contrast to the previously published books on the life and work of Mikao Usui, in which I hardly found anything in common between the described techniques and my own practice of the system, I felt a certain resonance between the contents of his teachings and my own practice in this book about Dr. Hayashi. I also had some "aha" experiences in terms of the origin of certain techniques and customs of *Usui Shiki Ryoho,* the Reiki system that I practice today.

So I recognized *Ketsueki Kokan,* a blood-circulation technique taught by Dr. Hayashi, as the origin of the "Energy Stroke," which I had learned as the completion of a treatment from my teacher, Paul Mitchell. Furthermore, the subdivision of the Third Degree into *Shihan Kaku* (teacher's assistant) and *Shihan* (teacher) reminded me of the custom within *Usui Shiki Ryoho* of giving the title of "Master Candidates" to students who are in the Master training. I had already been allowed to experience the *Reiki-Mawashi* that Tadao Yamaguchi describes in the book—everyone sits in a circle

43

and places their hands on the person sitting in front of them in order to feel the circulating Reiki energy—at some of the large Reiki meetings in Gersfeld, Germany, and this had touched me deeply each time.

In addition, this first book about Dr. Hayashi showed completely new facets of his personality and his work. Before then, the books by Fran Brown and Helen J. Haberly[21], two students of Hawayo Takata, describing the life and work of Mrs. Takata had been the only source about the person of Dr. Hayashi. But now there was finally a book dedicated exclusively to the life and work of Dr. Hayashi. Even if Dr. Hayashi played an important role in the books by Fran Brown and Helen Haberly as the teacher of Mrs. Takata, he appeared rather stylized throughout them. This certainly is one of the reasons why he has always remained something like the "unfamiliar great figure" within the Usui System of Reiki for many people. I had always seen Dr. Hayashi as a type of governor for Mikao Usui who preserved the system during a brief period before he placed it in the hands of Mrs. Takata, who then caused it to fully blossom. In view of the new situation revealed in the sources, it becomes increasingly clear that Dr. Hayashi himself had a decisive effect on the system before he handed it over to Mrs. Takata in 1938 on Hawaii.

A Shoden-Seminar with Dr. Hayashi

Based on the memories of Chiyoko Yamaguchi, who participated in a *Shoden* seminar with Dr. Hayashi in 1935[22], a typical seminar day looked like this: The room in which the seminar took place was first somewhat darkened. The participants sat in the classical Japanese style of sitting, *Seiza,* which is kneeling on the floor. They held their hands in the *Gassho* posture, the palms placed together in front of the hearts while they received their first *Reiju* energy transmission, which was carried out by Dr. Hayashi's students. Afterward, Dr. Hayashi entered the room. Under his instruction, the Principles were recited together. Finally, the room was completely darkened. Now the actual *Reiju* energy transmission took place, performed by Dr. Hayashi personally. As he did this, he dedicated about five minutes to each of the participants. He recited the poetry of the Meiji Emperor during the initiation ritual.

All of the participants met together afterward and formed a Reiki *Mawashi* to circulate the energy. This was followed later by Dr. Hayashi's lecture, in easily understandable terms, on topics related to Reiki. Examples of these are the natural cleansing process that Reiki produces in people, the phenomenon of the initial worsening, or the personal responsibility that the individual bears within the society. Dr. Hayashi apparently used anatomic diagrams to explain the functions of the individual organs. Reiki was finally practiced in the afternoon using 40-centimeter (16-inch) high rattan loungers and futons placed on the floor. During this activity, Dr. Hayashi also gave explanations on how to use the techniques with which the participants could develop their intuition. These also included the technique of *Byosen,* which was certainly very close to his heart as a physician.

The Technique of Byosen

Even during Mikao Usui's time, the technique of *Byosen* was the most important foundation for treating people with Reiki.[23] *Byosen* means something like "disease frequency." The technique of *Byosen* involves finding the source of the vibration radiating the disease within the body of the person to be treated and keeping the hands there until the disease frequency changes or disappears. Hiroko Kasahara describes it in the following words:

"Byosen can be found at the cause or source of the disease, and not always where the pain or the symptom occurs. The head is usually also treated since it contains the center for the powers of self-healing.

45

But the usual approach is not to perform a full-body treatment but a specific treatment."[24]

Within the rank system according to Mikao Usui, which Dr. Hayashi kept, only those who had achieved a certain competence in the technique of *Byosen* rose into the next rank, namely from the Sixth Rank into the Fifth Rank. The Fourth Rank was only bestowed upon those whose hands were intuitively led to *Byosen* right away. The Third Rank, which was the precondition for learning the Second Degree, was only given to those who, according to the teacher's assessment, had reached a certain high level in their treatments in terms of their healing powers.[25]

Seen in this light, both Mikao Usui and Dr. Hayashi taught a very intuitive way of using Reiki. According to this report, only those students whose intuition was not developed strongly enough followed the treatment plan for their hand positions. The plan was probably created especially for this purpose by Usui[26] (cf. pg. 156). We can assume that at the time of Dr. Hayashi, the treatment plan that he developed (cf. pg. 160) was also used for this purpose.

Further information on the technique of *Byosen* can be found in *The Hayashi Reiki Manual* by Frank Arjava Petter and Tadao Yamaguchi[27]. There is a simple exercise on page 48 for becoming familiar with *Byosen,* as instructed by Frank Arjava Petter[28].

Great Success

According to a number of different sources, Dr. Hayashi was very successful on the whole with his Reiki seminars. For example, Frank Arjava Petter writes: "Dr. Hayashi became quite famous in his day and the size of his group actually greatly exceeded the original *Usui Reiki Ryoho Gakkai.*"[29] Many of his students came from the upper classes of society and were artists, writers, or entrepreneurs, for example.[30] This may have primarily been related to the high costs of the seminars. Dr. Hayashi, as Tadao Yamaguchi writes, supposedly charged 50 Yen for the First Degree, *Shoden;* this corresponds to a current amount of several thousand US-Dollars.[31]

In a newspaper article from the year 1928, which is printed in full length in *The Hayashi Reiki Manual,* a Mr. Matsui reports on his experiences with Dr. Hayashi and Reiki. Here is an excerpt from it:

"A mutual friend introduced me to Mr. Hayashi and I decided to learn Reiki from him. I paid a fortune to be attuned. There are different levels of study, *Shoden* and *Okuden* are two of them. I have learned *Shoden* level but I am still a beginner so as yet I haven't been ready to move to the *Okuden* level. I don't know all the details yet but I have noticed that there seems to be a hierarchy among the students. I find it quite interesting that these well-intentioned people, who are too modest but brag about the wonderful things they can do, have created such a hierarchy and charge so much money for giving initiations. However I do believe that they should be allowed to maintain their own interests. But I feel so frustrated that I am not free to talk about the details of the initiation and treatment. In my opinion it is a great loss for everyone."[32]

A New Student

One day near the end of 1935[33], a young woman from Hawaii appeared at Dr. Hayashi's Reiki clinic. She was the child of Japanese parents who had immigrated during the previous century. Her name was Hawayo Takata. She first requested to receive Reiki treatments in order to heal her severe abdominal ailments—she had a tumor and gallstones. Later, after her ailments had been completely healed through Reiki, she absolutely wanted to learn the First Degree. However, this was not possible at first because the rules of the *Hayashi Reiki Kenkyukai* said that no foreigners were permitted.

Byosen Partner Exercise
As instructed by Frank Arjava Petter

To get a clear feeling for the Byosen, practice the following exercise with a partner:

1. Place one hand on your own knee or thigh (if they are healthy, otherwise choose another non-tense part of the body) and the other one on the shoulder of your partner in front of you.

Feel the difference of perception in each of your hands. The hand resting on your knee will feel "normal." It may feel warm and relaxed, radiating energy in a calm and even manner, the same way you perceive a "normal" pulse. The other hand will feel the tension in your partner's shoulders and upper back. Since most of us lead rather sedentary lives and have acquired poor posture, we have tense shoulders. Through this exercise, you will be able to recognize the difference between a relaxed and harmonious part of the body and a tense one.

2. Now hold both of your hands on your partner's shoulders for a few minutes and give him or her Reiki.

The sensation of the Byosen will become less intense as you go along. If the tension is not very pronounced in the first place, it may even vanish all together and your partner will be enveloped in warmth and relaxation.

3. Now switch your hands. Place the hand that was on your knee or your thigh (or another part of the body that was not tense) at the beginning on your partner's shoulder. And place the other hand that had been on your partner's shoulder on a part of your body that is not tense.

The sensitivity of your right and left hands is likely to be slightly different. It is not a question of being right or left-handed. For some right-handers, the left hand is more sensitive than the right and vice versa. Experiment and find out for yourself: is it the Byosen that you feel or is it the energy in your own hand?

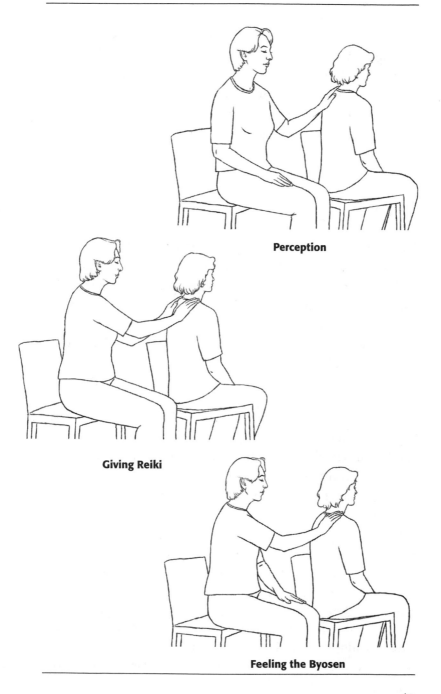

Perception

Giving Reiki

Feeling the Byosen

Since Mrs. Takata insisted and presented good reasons for her wish, in addition to a letter of recommendation from a well-known physician, there were deliberations about how her request could be filled without violating the rules of the society.[34] Helen Haberly, one of Mrs. Takata's students, wrote the following: "Dr. Hayashi called the directors of the association to a meeting where this appeal was read. It was decided to allow Mrs. Takata to become an honorary member, a special privilege which would permit her to take the Reiki Healing lessons; and when the next class was offered, she was allowed to enroll."[35]

As Helen Haberly also writes, Mrs. Takata stayed in Tokyo for about one year after learning the First Degree to continue her training in Reiki. Dr. Hayashi allowed her to work during the mornings in the clinic, and she had house visits to go on in the afternoons. After she had adequately developed her intuitive abilities, she was allowed to enroll in the *Okuden* Seminar. In 1937, she received the initiation into the Second Degree.

"Having completed her training with Dr. Hayashi, Mrs. Takata returned home to Kauai in the summer of 1937. A few weeks later Dr. Hayashi and his daughter arrived to spend six months visiting and helping establish Reiki Healing in Hawaii. It was decided that Honolulu was the best place to offer classes, so they rented two hotel bungalows and began offering free lectures and demonstrations of this healing art. The editor of the Japanese newspaper was very helpful, publishing pictures and articles in support of Reiki Healing, so within a short time it was well received by the people. Soon they rented a larger hall where lectures and classes were given by Dr. Hayashi, with Mrs. Takata assisting."[36]

In view of this development, we can probably assume that a very special connection had developed between Dr. Hayashi and Mrs. Takata. After all, Dr. Hayashi traveled to Hawaii and stayed for a good half year, leaving Japan and his Reiki clinic, as well as his numerous students for a considerable amount of time. In February of 1938, it was finally time for him to go back to Tokyo:

"His friends gave a banquet in his honor, where they presented him with many gifts and mementos of his visit to Hawaii, expressions of gratitude for allowing Reiki Healing to be taken beyond Japan. He used this occasion to announce publicly that Mrs. Takata was a Reiki Master, chosen for this work because she had passed many tests and proved herself worthy; so it was widely known that she was qualified to continue the Reiki Healing practice and to teach classes in Hawaii."[37]

Dr. Hayashi's Death

Back in Japan, Dr. Hayashi only had about two years left until his death in May of 1940. There are many legends about the way in which he died. Tadao Yamaguchi writes the following: "How Hayashi Sensei died is thought to be a mystery but the facts are known. A relative of Chiyoko Yamaguchi heard the story directly from Chie Hayashi, Hayashi Sensei's wife. The war was becoming increasingly fierce and as an ex-serviceman Hayashi Sensei was expecting imminent call up for military service. Having become a dedicated practitioner of Reiki under the instruction of Usui Sensei it was impossible for him to participate in the war as a military officer, even as a medical officer. He knew that he would not be permitted to provide Reiki treatments on the battlefield and that he would have to practice conventional medicine with which he did not agree. Because of this travel to Hawaii Hayashi Sensei was also suspected of being a spy. He was faced with the impossible choice between going to war or being imprisoned and executed. He decided to die with dignity and ended his life himself in the presence of his wife and some of his students."[38]

51

Chujiro Hayashi passed away on May 11, 1940 at his country house in Atami.[39] At the time of his death, there were 13 people who he had initiated into the Third Degree *(Shinpiden)*. These included two women: his wife, Chie Hayashi, and Hawayo Takata.[40]

While Mrs. Takata continued Dr. Hayashi's work on Hawaii and the American mainland as his successor, his wife, Mrs. Chie Hayashi, attempted to carry on the work in Japan. She took over the direction of the *Hayashi Reiki Kenkyukai* and traveled throughout Japan to hold seminars and visit the various branches of the society. As we can read from Tadao Yamaguchi, he and his mother heard an interesting story from a man whose wife had participated in the seminars by Mrs. Hayashi. According to him, at a Buddhist memorial ceremony for Dr. Hayashi that took place in 1952 in Daishoji, a lady called Mrs. Takata came from Hawaii to pay her respects: "Chie Hayashi Sensei asked her to come to Japan permanently and to take over *Hayashi Reiki Kenkyukai* but she declined. It had been too long since she had learned Reiki from Hayashi Sensei and she had already started to alter and popularize it in Hawaii. It is not certain how seriously Mrs. Hayashi tried to convince Mrs. Takata to accept her proposal but she often lamented the difficulties in finding suitable successors."[41]

After Chie Hayashi's death, there was no one left to take over the *Hayashi Reiki Kenkyukai*. "Although Mr. and Mrs. Hayashi had two children (a son and a daughter), they decided against Reiki since they had suffered due to their parents constantly traveling because of Reiki."[42]

Further Developments

Before I continue, I would like to expressly thank Hiroko Kasahara, Frank Arjava Petter, and Tadao Yamaguchi for letting me quote so many passages from their works. Thanks to their research and contacts in Japan, we have been able to acquire an initial overview of the early phase of the Usui System's history. The following information about Toshihiro Eguchi and Kaiji Tomita comes primarily from the article "Reiki in Japan" by Hiroko Kasahara, which appeared in the *Reiki Magazin*.[43]

Toshihiro Eguchi

Toshihiro Eguchi learned the Reiki method of healing between 1925 and 1927. According to the research of Frank Arjava Petter and Dave King, he was among the circle of people initiated by Usui into Shinpiden, the Third Degree. After he left the *Usui Reiki Ryoho Gakkai,* which was apparently in protest against its high membership fees, he founded the *Tenohira Ryoji Kenkyukai* (Research Society for the Treatment with Palms). About 500,000 people reportedly learned this form of the Reiki healing method that developed within this society in Japan during the following years.

Kaiji Tomita

Kaiji Tomita probably learned the Reiki method of healing in 1925. Unfortunately, we do not know from whom he learned it. (At this time, some of the teachers initiated by Usui into this method had apparently already begun to teach it.) Kaiji Tomita established the *Tomita-Ryu Teate Ryoho,* which means something like the "Tomita System for the Healing Method through Laying On Hands." Seven years after Mikao Usui's death, Tomita published a book in which he described his methods of Reiki. This book has now been rediscovered and was reprinted in Japan in 1999. About 200,000 people in Japan have supposedly learned the system of Reiki founded by Tomita.

In addition to the *Usui Reiki Ryoho Gakkai,* Dr. Hayashi, Toshihiro Eguchi, and Kaiji Tomita, there were apparently other people from

53

Mikao Usui's circle who continued to develop the Reiki method of healing after Usui's death by founding their own societies or developing their own methods. Up until the Second World War, the number of those who were practicing a healing method through laying on hands had reportedly increased to approximately one million. However, as mentioned above, there was a radical change of values after the Second World War in Japan that resulted in an almost total extinction of interest in the traditional methods of healing, among other consequences. This also meant that there was no longer any significant dissemination of the Reiki healing method after 1945 in Japan.

3. Bridges into the West
The Usui System in a New Garment

The Usui System of Reiki probably found its way into the Western world on two different paths. Both of them led over Dr. Hayashi and, in the following time, through two of his students. While his official successor, Hawayo Takata, brought the Usui System of Reiki into the West through Hawaii, another student of Dr. Hayashi, the Zen monk Takeuchi, reportedly developed a meditative variation of the system, which later also reached the West. However, it was Hawayo Takata who played the central role in spreading the Usui System of Reiki throughout the world. Her work laid the foundation for the Usui System becoming an internationally wide-spread healing method during the course of the 20th Century. From Paul Mitchell's perspective, this process is described in the following way:

"Dr. Hayashi went beyond the boundaries of tradition to teach Reiki outside of Japan, even though he taught only Japanese people in Hawaii. Mrs. Takata went beyond those boundaries by teaching non-Japanese people. This was a momentous decision. In effect, it made the practice available to the world. In doing this, she translated and interpreted the system for a universal culture, the human culture. To do this she stripped away any religious aspects that may have been part of the practice as well as Japanese cultural aspects. She simplified the practice to give us a universal human healing art true to the spirit of Dr. Usui."[1]

In addition to Hawayo Takata, there was reportedly another student of Dr. Hayashi through whom one lineage of the Usui System leads to the West. As we read in an article by Gordon Bell[2], this was the

55

monk Takeuchi, the abbot of a Zen temple. He reportedly received a series of meditations from Dr. Hayashi, in addition to the usual contents of the *Reiki Ryoho*. These are supposedly the meditations that Usui practiced on Mount Kurama. The monk Takeuchi apparently passed on this knowledge to his student Seiji Takamori, among other people, and the Usui System ultimately reached the West through this lineage. The distinguishing characteristic of this lineage is that the lineage bearers have constantly deepened the meditative aspect of the Usui System and merged it with Tibetan-Buddhist practices, in which they recognized commonalities with the Usui System. In the early 1970s, Seiji Takamori reportedly also met with Hawayo Takata on his journey through the USA.

Hawayo Takata

Hawayo Takata was born on Christmas Eve of the year 1900 on Hawaii as the third child of a young Japanese couple. As depicted in the books of Helen J. Haberly and Fran Brown, she had a difficult youth. Even as a 13-year-old, she had to work in the sugar-cane fields during summer vacation to earn money for her family. In addition, she had other jobs to do.[3] Fran Brown describes her situation at that time in the following words: "She had finished the American school, but she continued in the Japanese school from six to eight in the morning. Then she walked the seven miles to her job at the soda fountain. In her spare time, she did filing in the office of the general store."[4]

The young Hawayo soon experienced a considerable improvement of her situation: She found work in the household of an "elegant lady" who lived in a mansion in the colonial style. With time, she moved up into the position of head housekeeper and became the supervisor to about 20 employees.[5] "This lady also had in her employ a young Japanese accountant whom she felt needed a wife. And she hoped he and Hawayo would like each other. They did.

On March 10, 1917, Saichi Takata and Hawayo Kawamura were married, and they were very happy together. They had two little girls, the first one being born on the elegant lady's birthday, much to her delight. Then Saichi became ill and went to Tokyo to the Maeda Clinic for treatment. In 1930, at the age of 34, he died of lung cancer. This was a great shock and terrible loss to the family and community (...)."[6]

Unfortunately, Hawayo Takata was also not spared of additional blows of fate. After the death of her husband, she worked very hard to financially provide for her family. As a result, she became very ill, had a nervous breakdown, and ultimately developed a painful abdominal condition. It turned out that she had a uterine tumor that had to be operated. Moreover, one of her sisters died at this time of tetanus. All of this happened in 1935, while her parents had returned to Japan to visit for a year, which was the first time since their emigration in 1895. Hawayo Takata felt that she could not tell her parents the news of her sister's death in a letter and decided to travel to Japan to give it to them personally. At this opportunity, she also planned to have an operation on the tumor.[7]

After she had arrived in Japan and had given her parents the sad news of her sister's death, she went to Tokyo and entered the Madea Clinic. As Mrs. Takata liked to say later in her Reiki classes, she was already laying on the operating table when she heard a voice that said: "The operation is not necessary." When the doctor came in, she asked him because of this experience whether there might be another possibility for her than the planned operation. The doctor thought about it for a moment and then recommended that she go to Dr. Hayashi's Reiki clinic. Mrs. Takata went on her way and discovered, as we know, Reiki.

The "Soul of the Usui System"

According to everything that we know about Hawayo Takata today, she appears to have been a very impressive personality. Many people who personally knew her still talk about her with great reverence in their voices and convey the feeling that Mrs. Takata remains an authority for them. The impression that I received from the conversations with the Masters initiated by Mrs. Takata, including Phyllis Furumoto, Wanja Twan and Paul Mitchell, Takata embodied what we could call the "soul of the Usui System" with her whole being. When she began to initiate Reiki Masters in the mid-1970s, she could already look back at almost 40 years of practicing the system. During this time, she had continually dedicated her life to the practice and teachings of the system. As far as I know, up to now no other lineage bearer in the history of the Usui System is able to look back on such long years of experience with the Usui System of Reiki.

In order to get an impression of Mrs. Takata as a person and her appearance it makes sense to read the words of someone who knew her personally. In her book *In the Light of a Distant Star*, Wanja Twan, who was initiated into all three degrees of the Usui System during the 1970s by Hawayo Takata, writes about her first encounter with her teacher on the first seminar day of a First Degree seminar at the home of Barbara Brown:

"Since we were late, we drove at high speed in an old pick-up, and within twenty minutes I stood in front of Barbara Brown's door, knocking. 'Come in', I heard a voice call from somewhere inside the house. I opened the door, my eyes fell on a woman coming down a stairway just in front of me. She was a beautiful older Japanese woman with shiny, light grey hair and dressed in a long, blue Hawaiian dress with exotic flowers. 'I knew you would come,' she said as she looked at me with a wink in her eye.

I followed Takata into the living room where Barbara bade me welcome and gestured for me to sit down together with the other seven or eight people who had gathered for the course. In the centre of the room stood a table made of a piece of plywood laid across two sawhorses and covered with a thin foamie and a sleeping bag with a nice, crocheted zig-zag afghan at the foot.

Takata greeted everyone politely and made a gesture, bidding someone to come forward and lay down on the table. A man came forward and someone steadied the piece of plywood as he lay down on the table. Takata sat down on a chair opposite us, put her hands on the man's midriff and proceeded to talk.

She told us the story of Reiki, how it first had been revealed, how she had come in contact with it and had subsequently learned it and the experiences she had had over the forty years that she had practiced it. I listened intently as I watched her hands move over the man's body in a set pattern, yet lingering longer in some places where the hands' innate knowledge seemed to guide them with great professionalism. I watched her occasionally glance down at his body as if she was looking at it with x-ray vision in a kind way. A realization came over me that I was witnessing something very special and remarkable, that I was part of an event of some magnitude.

Her talk lasted about an hour. The man on the table had been replaced with a woman, who got up from the table a bit dazedly when we were asked to go to an upstairs room a few at a time for the initiations. I was among the last and went up with a young man. Takata motioned for us to sit down on two chairs that were placed in the middle of the room, close our eyes and put our hands up in a prayer-like fashion. I felt her presence behind me and had a feeling that she was praying over me. It caused my head to tingle and I felt warmth at the top of my head. I also felt as if I was a creaky, rusty old oil lamp, and that she was making the lid open up, so I could be filled up with oil and light up like a bright new light.

On the way downstairs I started to wonder at it all—it had happened so quickly—how did she do the initiations, how did she know that I was going to come and how was all this going to affect my life? I sat down on the sofa in the living room and by now Barbara's husband had lit a lovely fire in the fireplace that was crackling in the soft, quiet atmosphere of the room where we all sat silently waiting for Takata to come down. I looked out the windows at the darkening skies with the trees silhouetted against it. The stars were just starting to come out. I heard Barbara setting teacups on a tray in the kitchen. I brought my gaze into the room, resting it for a while on some wild flowers in a vase on the table, then let it wander to a large petitpoint picture on the wall above the fireplace. The colours and threads in it were beautifully, softly aged; the picture portrayed a man with a falcon on his arm and a horse in the background. In the foreground lay a spear and a glove thrown down—a thought ran through my head, 'The glove is thrown—do you accept the challenge?' In that moment Takata entered the room, and we had tea."[8]

The Reiki History According to Hawayo Takata

After increasing information about the origins of the Usui System (including the life and work of Mikao Usui and Dr. Hayashi) had reached the public in recent years, there were some posthumous accusations against Hawayo Takata and/or her version of the history of the Usui System. These claimed that she had "Christianized" the history by making Mikao Usui into a Christian priest and also that further inaccuracies ranging up to the version of the history passed orally from Master to Master had become apparent. However, it should be stressed that Takata's version of the history—with the exception of the fact that Mikao Usui was not a Christian priest—still remains correct in its main points. Perhaps Mikao Usui was never enrolled at the University of Chicago, but it is certain, as stated by the memorial-stone inscription, that he traveled to America and engaged in extensive studies in diverse areas of knowledge (cf. pg. 19/26). Perhaps he also never lived in an impoverished neighborhood, but it is considered certain that he took care of people in need, especially after the terrible earthquake in Tokyo in 1923 (cf. pg. 29). And even if he was not a Christian priest, he was at least familiar with the Christian ideas, as reported in the memorial-stone inscription (cf. pg. 26).

I think that it was Hawayo Takata's great service to have brought the Usui System into a form in which it was finally able to spread throughout the world. It is estimated that more than 90 percent of all practitioners throughout the world have learned a form of the Usui System that is essentially based on the form shaped by Hawayo Takata. Within the historical circumstances in which Mrs. Takata began to teach the Usui System—in the 1940s and 1950s in the USA, an era that was characterized by mistrust against other world views—she apparently thought it made sense to present the history of the Usui System in a way that we could call "legendary." It is my feeling that she did this based on a pure motivation, with the goal of teaching as many people as possible an appreciation for the Usui System of Reiki while still remaining connected with her teacher, Dr. Hayashi, in a deep sense of esteem.

The Usui System on Hawaii

After Hawayo Takata received the initiation into the First Degree in 1936 from Dr. Hayashi, as the first foreigner in the history of the Usui System, she was very enthusiastic about the new practice that she had learned. As a result, she remained in Tokyo for about a year to deepen her connection with Dr. Hayashi and prepare herself for the Second Degree. Helen Haberly has written about this period:

"Takata moved to the Hayashi home, accepting their invitation to live with them while she learned to be a Reiki Healing practitioner.

When the first patients started arriving at seven each morning, Mrs. Takata was in the clinic with the other sixteen practitioners, where for five hours there was not an idle moment. The afternoons were used for house calls, sometimes requiring a train ride of two or three hours out into the country and back again after treating the patient. Following her evening meal she gave the report of her afternoon's activities to Dr. Hayashi and his family. This was her daily routine for one year, with every day devoted to the practice of Reiki Healing."[9]

As Fran Brown writes, Dr. Hayashi was apparently inspired by Hawayo Takata's lively nature: "Dr. Hayashi was always amused when Takata asked questions. Because it was so foreign to the ways of the Japanese ladies who never dared to question anything, he considered the direct wanting-to-know quality of curiosity which was so much a part of Takata as 'American democracy in action'."[10]

After Mrs. Takata had received the initiation into the Second Degree in 1937, she returned to Hawaii after almost two continuous years of living in Japan. Just a few weeks later, Dr. Hayashi came to Hawaii for six months and held Reiki seminars with her there.[11] Before he left again in February of 1938, he used the occasion of a banquet that took place in his honor to announce that Mrs. Takata was now a Reiki Master. As he did so, he gave her a notarized certificate in which he attested that she was the only Reiki Master in the United States at this time and that she was empowered by him to confer "the power of Reiki on others."[12]

In this certificate, Dr. Hayashi used three different names for the Usui System of Reiki: "The Usui System of Reiki Healing," "The Usui System of Drugless Healing," and "Dr. Usui's Reiki System of Healing."[13] Furthermore, he spoke of himself and Mrs. Takata as "Reiki Masters." From this time on, this phrase entered into the terminology of the Usui System to describe those who had been initiated into the Third Degree, *Shinpiden.*

In the following period of time, Mrs. Takata began to spread the Usui System on the Hawaiian Islands. Although she had originally taught in Honolulu together with Dr. Hayashi, she shifted the focus of her work, as Helen Haberly writes,[14] to the main island of Hawaii. In 1938, she held the first seminars there in Kamuela, and starting in 1939 she also taught in Kona and Pahoa. During this time she received an invitation to take a vacation in Hilo, which came from two ladies who were interested in Reiki. She accepted their invitation, and, during this vacation, coincidentally found a suitable house that she wanted to use as a Reiki center and could also afford since monthly installments were possible. She soon moved from Honolulu to the Island of Hawaii and opened her Reiki center there. She gave many treatments, and had very successful results, in addition to holding numerous seminars at her new Reiki center in Hilo and on the entire island.

At the beginning of 1940, she had a dream that caused her to travel back to Japan and visit Dr. Hayashi. As she ultimately discovered, Dr. Hayashi had decided to prematurely end his life because of the difficult situation he had gotten into due to the pending participation of Japan in the Second World War (cf. pg. 51). He reportedly made this "transition" in the presence of his wife, Hawayo Takata, and some of his other close students at his country house in Atami. Shortly before, he apparently named Mrs. Takata officially as his successor. Dr. Hayashi's corpse was brought to Tokyo, "where he lay in state at the Reiki Center and was visited by many people from all over Japan who came to express their respect for this great man. For a full week this continued and his body showed no signs of deterioration."[15]

A short time later, Mrs. Takata returned to Hawaii. Here she continued her healing work based on Dr. Hayashi, while his wife, Chie Hayashi, endeavored to carry on his work in Japan.

Wondrous Stories

If we believe the many stories about Mrs. Takata that Fran Brown and Helen J. Haberly describe in their books[16], Takata had proved to have many healing successes with her patients over time. No matter whether it was a headache, heart attack, or ulcers: She could almost always help. So a great portion of her healing work consisted of Reiki treatments. One day she had an amazing experience at a funeral celebration to which she had been invited by a Japanese-American family. In the words of Mrs. Takata:

"I felt out of place. I didn't know a soul, and so I said to myself, 'My position is in the bedroom with the dead.' So I stood by the bed, and placed a chair there, and put my hands on the dead body, on the solar plexus. I was trying to kill time; I didn't know what else to do. I was also trying to comfort the daughter, who was there crying and screaming and asking for forgiveness. By 9:30 I had had my hands on the body for about an hour and a half. I gave the dead body Reiki, Reiki, Reiki. That was all I could do. I felt very comfortable about it, because I was doing something and not sitting idly by. I couldn't go into the room where they were preparing the funeral, I couldn't go into the kitchen where they were cooking, and so I sat in the bedroom with my hand on the dead body. And, do you know? At 9:30 she woke up. All of a sudden, she looked at me, and I looked at her, and I said, 'Mama, you are up.' She said, 'Ah, yes, ah.' I felt very strange and awkward. I didn't know what to say, but I said, 'What can I do for you?' She said, 'I'm hungry!' I said, 'Good idea!' She said, 'I haven't eaten for three days and I'm very hungry.' She remembered that! I foolishly asked her, 'What would you like to eat?' She said, 'A bowl of hot *sai min (sai min* is

Chinese noodle soup that we usually eat for snack or for lunch). So I said, 'OK, you shall have it.'"[17]

After Mrs. Takata coincidentally brought back the supposedly dead woman by means of Reiki, the funeral was quickly cancelled. A bowl of the hot sai min soup was brought for the presumably dead relative, and the family was confronted with the unbelievable situation that she had come back to life. She continued to enjoy the best of health for many years to come.

The years passed, and "after almost a decade of success with her healing center at Hilo, Mrs. Takata returned to Honolulu where she made her home for the next thirty years, and there she continued her work with Reiki Healing. Maintaining a treatment center in this city, she also traveled among the islands, conducting classes as usual and making an occasional trip to the American mainland; but the greater emphasis was in Hawaii where she had hundreds of Reiki Healing students.

During the fall of 1973 she was invited to teach a large group on an island off the coast of Washington state, and this was the start of seven very busy years. As the requests for classes began to fill her schedule, she traveled to the Pacific Coast, the Mid-West, East, South, Southwest and into Canada; and with these demands, there was less and less time for the clinic work. The teaching had become a full-time occupation."[18]

Takata's Teachings

Takata's way of teaching was apparently very simple and direct. Everyone who knew her personally emphasizes that she did not want the course participants to take notes. She demanded the undivided attention of all the participants when she spoke or demonstrated something:

"No notes. I want your eyes on my hands. I will only do this once. Watch what I do and remember it. If you are looking at your book, you don't see my hands."[19]

In an interview that she gave in 1973, she described the contents of her seminars as follows:

"In the first lesson, I explain the universal life force, what it is, and I explain the workings of cosmic energy and how to make contact. I maneuver it so that they have it. So far I have never made a mistake. They come to the lecture and they get it from me. The second lesson is how to use it. This is a demonstration of applying the healing from the neck up, eye, ear, nose, mouth, glands of the neck. I teach them how. The third day I teach them how to treat the organs in the front of the body. The fourth day I teach them how to apply it to the back. I take the body in sections so they don't forget or they'd get mixed up. The last day is the mental and spiritual lecture—mental attitudes, meditation. When they acquire this Reiki it is a complete treatment for the physical body, the mental and the spiritual being."[20]

However, the example of the process described here, which stretches over four to five days, only developed through the course of time. It appears that Takata's seminars were less extensive in the early days, at least according to the memory of Toshiko Takaezo, who participated in one of her First Degree seminars on Hawaii in 1949 or 1950:

"It was a medium-sized class, in a living room, for one or two evenings only. She did not talk or explain much. She was very direct, and went immediately to the core, right into the treatment. As far as I remember now, she didn't tell us much of anything about her teachers. No story, just doing Reiki. All the history and her experiences, I read about these only years later, from Helen Haberly's book."[21]

It becomes clear here that even in Takata's early years as a Reiki Master, her directness was a very special trait of her personal teaching style. One of the themes that she, like Dr. Hayashi, enjoyed discussing and frequently talked about were the physical reactions that Reiki can trigger in people. Fran Brown writes the following on this subject:

"Each time Takata taught a class she would talk about 'reactions.' When Reiki treatments are begun, a great change takes place, and all the energy bodies are affected as the physical body begins to detoxify itself. The cleansing of the physical body starts as the vitalized organs begin to return to normal. This is called 'reaction,' and after this is finished, the body is much more normal and is then able to heal itself. The reaction shows whether the healing is moving forward."[22]

While she continued this aspect of Dr. Hayashi's teachings, she completely dispensed with another essential element of the teachings of Dr. Hayashi and Mikao Usui: the poems of the Meiji Emperor (cf. pg. 31–32). These had probably disappeared from the system since the transference of the Usui System from Japan to Hawaii (or also since Takata had begun teaching non-Japanese), which may be related to the fact that the essence of this poetry can hardly be translated into English in the appropriate way. At the same time, Mrs. Takata preserved another important component of the teachings of Dr. Hayashi and Mikao Usui, namely the Reiki Principles as a significant element of the system. Here is a formulation of the Principles in Old English, as written by Hawayo Takata:

> "Just for today—Thou shalt not anger.
> Just for today—Thou shalt not worry.
> Thou shalt be grateful for the many blessings.
> Earn thy livlihood with honest labour.
> Be kind to thy neighbors."[23]

The recitation of the Principles, which was still very customary during the time of Mikao Usui and Dr. Hayashi[24], stopped completely with Takata. At the same time, it appears she had her very own way of conveying the Principles to the participants of her courses. In the words of her granddaughter and successor, Phyllis Furumoto:

"When Takata taught the precepts in her classes, she just said them. They weren't written down. Most people wrote them down, but she didn't present anything or hand them out. She would just say, 'This is what we live by…' That was it. You heard them once. If you didn't get them, too bad. She didn't worry about it."[25]

Through Mrs. Takata's personal teaching style, the principle of the oral tradition became increasingly important. As many seminar participants unanimously report, she did not hand out any paperwork. Instead, the transmission of information was concentrated solely on situations in which the student encountered her personally, either within the scope of a seminar or elsewhere. In terms of the contents that Mrs. Takata imparted in her seminars over the course of the years, they were basically identical in their essence. However, she apparently always found new ways to convey these contents in keeping with the respective participant structure of the seminars. For example, Helen Haberly has written the following on this topic:

"As a teacher, she spoke simply and with power: 'This is the way you do Reiki!' Yet, those who participated in more than one class found that she adjusted her instruction for each group, never presenting the information in the same way twice. At times she would tell her students to start the treatment with the head; at other times she would tell them to start with the abdomen; or she might say it really did not matter where they started so long as the complete treatment was given. She encouraged them to develop their intuitive 'feel' for

Reiki Healing and to do what seemed right for them individually, while observing the basic hand placements which she taught."[26]

Daily Self-Treatment

With the teachings of Mrs. Takata, the daily self-treatment became the focus of the practice in the Usui System. She taught a standard sequence of eight hand positions on the head and front side of the body for this purpose. This appears to be a fundamentally new element—neither the "Treatment Plans" according to Mikao Usui and Dr. Hayashi (cf. pgs. 156 ff.) nor other sources from this time contain references to a regular, daily self-treatment with Reiki.[27]

In addition, Mrs. Takata also taught a standard sequence of hand positions for the treatment of other people on the head, front side, and backside of the body. This was also apparently a new element since there are no references whatsoever to this in the treatment plans according to Mikao Usui and Dr. Hayashi or in other sources. (In the Treatment Plan according to Mikao Usui, just six head positions and one position for the treatment of the gastrointestinal area are mentioned under the heading "Basic Treatment for Specific Parts of the Body."[28] The Treatment Plan according to Dr. Hayashi published by Frank Arjava Petter, lists four head positions. According to a note, which appears to come from Frank Arjava Petter, these should be included as part of the treatment for any disease.[29] Bronwen and Frans Stiene write in *The Reiki Sourcebook* that Mikao Usui taught five head positions for the basic treatment of other people. He treated additional parts of the body in an intuitive way. The five head positions illustrated in this book are similar to the ones found as head positions in the treatment plans according to Mikao Usui and Dr. Hayashi.[30]

In keeping with this, it also appears that the basic sequences of the hand positions for self-treatment, as well as for the treatment of others, in the form that the majority of Reiki practitioners throughout the world have learned them, were created either by Mrs. Takata or by Dr. Hayashi (cf. pg. 162) before her. As Bronwen and Frans Stiene have written, Dave King (a Reiki Teacher who has researched the origins of the Usui System in Japan) discovered that Tatsumi, one of Dr. Hayashi's students, learned seven fundamental hand positions from Dr. Hayashi.[31] In terms of the Treatment Plan according to Dr. Hayashi, Mrs. Takata was supposedly also familiar with it.[32] Mrs. Takata was also apparently familiar with some of the meditation techniques that Mikao Usui taught, such as the *Hatsureiho* Meditation (cf. pg. 22) and the technique of *Reiju* Energy Transmission (cf. pg. 25). However, according to all of the information we have today, she very rarely passed on this knowledge for whatever reason.

Traveling

In the 1950s and 1960s, the focus of Mrs. Takata's life continued to be on the Hawaiian Islands. Yet, even back then she was already taking many trips to the American mainland and to other countries. In a portrait by the journalist Sally Hammond about Hawayo Takata, published in 1973 by Ballantine Books under the title of *We Are All Healers,* the author writes:

"Takata said that since reaching 61 she has not worked full-time. The last two years she's been traveling all over the world. 'But when I'm home, I work. I like teaching in groups of 10 or 12 because there's more competition,' she said briskly, 'and they can compare notes.' Her pupils come to her by word of mouth and she teaches many doctors and their wives, and a few celebrities. She names a famous American heiress but made me promise to keep it confidential."[33]

As we can read in the book by Mary McFadyen and the one by Bronwen and Frans Stiene, the mysterious heiress was probably Doris Duke, who was the richest woman in the world at that time. Mrs. Takata apparently traveled around the world with her and also worked with Hollywood celebrities like Danny Kaye. In addition, she initiated the well-known writer Aldous Huxley into the Usui System.[34]

In 1973, Mrs. Takata had initially made the decision to retire. As Fran Brown writes, Takata had had enough after 38 years of the teaching and healing. She had wanted to entrust this "wonderful Art" to a couple "who would bring youth and vigor to Reiki and carry on its traditions."[35] Instead, as we know, everything happened quite differently: In the very same year, she accepted an invitation to hold a seminar with more than 30 participants on an island off the coast of Washington State. This was the signal for a seven-year period filled with work, which lasted until her death in 1980.

First Master Initiations

In 1975, Mrs. Takata suffered a mild heart attack. John Harvey Gray writes: "At that time, she suddenly realized that she was the only person in the world to teach Reiki. And if she wanted Reiki to live after she died, she would need to make new Reiki Masters. I was in the first group of three persons who became Reiki Masters, the third in the Western world. That was in 1976."[36]

The other two Masters in this group were Virginia Samdahl and Ethel Lombardi. Of the two, Virginia Samdahl was the first female Reiki Master that Mrs. Takata had initiated. As we read in Bronwen and Frans Stiene's book, Mrs. Takata wrote in a letter that she sent in 1977 to her students that she had now found three Reiki Masters who should continue her work; these were Virginia Samdahl, Ethel Lombardi, and John Harvey Gray. On her 77th birthday, she then decided to finally retire.[37] But again, as we know, things happened quite differently: In the following three years she initiated 19 more Masters. There was no hint of retirement.

The Search for a Successor

Two of her Master students who had an especially distinctive relationship with Mrs. Takata in the years before her death were her granddaughter Phyllis Furumoto and Dr. Barbara Ray. Both received the initiation to become a Reiki Master from her in 1979.

As Phyllis Furumoto writes, she went on a longer trip in April of 1979 with her grandmother. At the beginning of it, she received the initiation into the Master Degree:

"I went back to Iowa to pick up my grandmother before we flew to Puerto Rico. We had three days. Takata sat me in a chair on the second day and said: 'Close your eyes, and sit like this!' I felt her move around me, and then I heard a clap. She said: 'Now you can work with me.'
I realized much later that she had a different picture of this 'work' than I did. I thought I'd be carrying suitcases, counting money, making sure she didn't get mugged on the street. But we came to the first Reiki class and she said, 'Now you're going to teach Reiki with me.' I said, 'What?!' She told me step by step everything to do, and I did it, and things worked. It was very strange."[38]

As Phyllis Furumoto writes in her article "Choosing Reiki,"[39] published in 2001 in the *Reiki Magazine International,* she grew up in a family in which, because of the circumstances, she came into contact with Reiki at a very early age. She apparently already received as a child the initiation into the First Degree, and later, at the end of her twenties, the initiation into the Second Degree.

There seemed to be a very special relationship between her and her grandmother: Takata told her what she expected from her and, after considerable reflection as to whether it was also right for her—which was probably the case most of the time—Phyllis accepted the respective challenge. As a result, she spent a great amount of time with her grandmother in the last two years before Takata's death and received extensive training. In describing another trip with her grandmother, that took place in the autumn of 1980, Phyllis Furumoto says:

"As I traveled with my grandmother, and now my Master, during the autumn of 1980, I paid more attention to the stories, to how people received them, and to what they seemed to learn from them. I was blessed to be present when three other Masters were initiated. I also had time alone with her to hear what she expected of me and what my life would be like. Though I did not always agree with her, what she asked of me, I gave. This involved a major shift in my belief system, as well as a large financial commitment. Shortly afterwards she left for the Seattle area and became ill. In December, she died. I was left with a strong connection between us that has grown into a precious relationship."[40]

Another one of the Masters initiated by Mrs. Takata who spent a great deal of time with her in 1979 and 1980 was Dr. Barbara Ray. With her academic background and her specialization in classical civilizations and languages,[41] she may have also shared some of her fundamental insights in terms of the background settings of the Usui System, with its symbols and ancient Japanese characters, with Mrs. Takata. If she engaged in this type of a reflection regarding her own decades of practice, it would have been something completely new for Mrs. Takata; something that perhaps fascinated her and opened up new worlds that had been undiscovered up to that point. She may also have hoped that the connection to Dr. Ray would also bring an appreciation by science for the Usui System of Reiki. Dr. Barbara Ray has written the following about her time with Mrs. Takata:

"During the last several years of her life, I had both the honor and the privilege of being with her in the privacy of her own home, in a small town in Iowa, for many weeks of intense study and training. In addition, in August 1980, I had the special honor of having her as a guest and teacher in my home in Atlanta for more than a month."[42]

Furthermore, we read that Dr. Ray and Mrs. Takata had begun "planning for an Association which was founded in 1980... she (Mrs. Takata, author's note) was present in Atlanta at the first-ever public meeting of The Reiki Association as its first and greatly honored guest. She spoke to the whole group and then spent much time graciously meeting personally with nearly all the two-hundred people attending."[43]

Acceleration

However, Dr. Barbara Ray and Phyllis Furumoto were not the only Masters initiated by Takata with whom she spent time during the last years of her life. It appears that she traveled extensively at that time through the USA and Canada, visited her students, held Reiki courses, and initiated many additional Masters, sometimes even without a larger interval of time between the Second Degree and the Master Degree or even a special training. For example, Paul Mitchell reports that he received the initiation into the First Degree in 1978 from Mrs. Takata. In 1979, having already been initiated into the Second Degree, he asked her whether she would initiate him into the Master Degree, while she was visiting him at his house:

"On that visit, I went with George Araki to speak with Mrs. Takata about mastery. That is something I never would have done on my own at that time; I wouldn't have had the courage. During that last visit, Mrs. Takata had another little talk with Susan (Paul Mitchell's wife, author's note), and said something like, 'Paul will do this for his life.' So that also gave me encouragement to be willing to ask her this. George and I told her that we wanted to teach Reiki some day, and she was willing to teach us. That was lovely and very affirming. We were initiated together the next day. And the day after that, I took Mrs. Takata to the airport. It was the last time that I saw her. We talked on the phone and corresponded, but she died before I was able to be with her again."[44]

Mary McFadyen received a similar spontaneous initiation into the Master Degree. A few weeks after she had received the initiation into the Second Degree from John Gray in July of 1980, she visited a seminar by Mrs. Takata in Oregon to get to know her and ask if she would initiate her into the Master Degree:

"I walked over to her and began to talk. I told her without pausing who I was, about my spiritual path, when I had received Reiki, about the Reiki that I had done and the experiences that I had had, and then I came to the big question: would she consider me as a potential Reiki Master? When I had finished speaking there was a moment of silence, and then Mrs. Takata said with great energy, 'Oh, we must start training you immediately!'"[45]

After some days of intensive time together, "in a whirlwind of activity, training, being with Mrs. Takata, and absorbing everything I could from her"[46], the paths of Mary McFadyen and Mrs. Takata parted again. At this point in time, Mary McFadyen's biggest dream, as she writes, had already been fulfilled: Mrs. Takata had initiated her as a Reiki Master.[47] Unfortunately, the intensive training that had been planned for the coming year never took place. There also were no more meetings between the two: Mrs. Takata passed away before the two could meet again.[48]

Training Periods

Yet, it appears that these types of "fast initiations" into the Master Degree were more of an exception for Mrs. Takata. Many of the other Masters who she initiated experienced much longer intervals of time between the individual initiation levels. For example, Shinobu Saito received the three Degrees in intervals of two years each: the First Degree in 1976, the Second Degree followed in 1978, and the initiation into the Master Degree finally took place in 1980.[49] Fran Brown received the First Degree from Mrs. Takata in 1973, the Second Degree in 1976 with John Gray (one of the Masters initiated by Mrs. Takata), and finally the initiation into the Master Degree from Mrs. Takata in 1979.[50]

While some of Mrs. Takata's Master students could only spend relatively little time with her because of the circumstances, others had more luck in this respect. For example, when someone organized a Reiki seminar for Mrs. Takata, it usually took place in the organizer's house and she lived there for the duration of the seminar. It appears that she cultivated a very personal connection with some of the Masters and students who she initiated in this way. Barbara Brown writes about a typical visit from Mrs. Takata with the following words:

"She lived with me a number of times, giving classes that I arranged for her. So I not only lived with her classes, I lived with her self. We went shopping with her, my husband drove her to stores, we went to cafés together, we did Reiki together, we sat together and talked."[51]

In Memoriam

As the stories by her students clearly illustrate over and over, Mrs. Takata appears to have been a very impressive woman with a unique presence. In her book *Reiki: Hawayo Takata's Story*, Helen J. Haberly summarizes the main qualities of her respected teacher into a portrait of several pages. Here are some excerpts:

"Even in the eighth decade of her life, Mrs. Takata was a very attractive woman, small boned, less than five feet in height, and weighing slightly over ninety pounds. Her motions were quick and decisive, and she moved with the ease of a young person, upright and graceful. (…) She truly cared for people, often putting their welfare and comfort before her own; and she offered treatment freely to those she met along the way, at times for only a few minutes. 'Better some Reiki than none at all,' she would say. (…) She lived quite simply, advocating a diet with many fresh vegetables and fruits, whole grains, fish and chicken, and although she would eat red meats, she did so sparingly. (…) Golfing, at which she was quite accomplished, was her favorite exercise, and when she was in Honolulu she walked to the golf course each morning to play. She liked to travel and especially enjoyed sightseeing in new areas she had not previously visited, often seeking out the local golf courses. (…) Those who knew her well realized she did not interpret the Spiritual Precept, 'Just for today, do not anger,' to mean that she should never anger. She had a healthy temper and at times would display it, but these times were few and involved only extreme conditions. When these did occur, she immediately responded, saying what needed to be said, doing what needed to be done to clear the air and restore balance. (…) She had a lively personality with the simplicity and open curiosity of a child, asking questions and exploring new ideas, ever probing and learning. She combined this simplicity with an insight that is found only in wisdom, so to those with whom she felt a close connection, she offered advice. (…) Along with her strength came an implacable quality where Reiki Healing was concerned. She allowed most of the foibles of humanity to flow by without comment, but she did not accept any nonsense in the discussion of Reiki Healing. She took her work very seriously, clarifying without hesitation the misconceptions held by another. When she shook her finger at someone, it emphasized her convictions gained through many years of experience, and there was no arguing with her on this subject—she was the authority and there was no mistaking it."[52]

The Gift of Reiki

While working on this book and reflecting on the correlations between Mrs. Takata's teachings, I sometimes asked myself the question: If Mrs. Takata were still alive today, what type of exercise or text would contribute to this book? I also directed this question to my teacher, Paul Mitchell. We thought about it for a while and then agreed that he would attempt to write an appropriate text in memory of Mrs. Takata. The result is below.

Hawayo Takata's Directives
In the words of Paul Mitchell

Mrs. Takata was very clear about the roles of teacher and student. Her role was to pass on the gift of Reiki and teach the practice. The student's role was to practice. Here is what she would say to students of Reiki.

Treat yourself every day. That means a full self-treatment.

Practice the Principles. That means live them.

Count your blessings. Gratitude is very important. Take time every day to be aware of all that you have to be grateful for.

Takata's Death

Above all, the last two years of Mrs. Takata's life seem to have been a whirlwind of activities and "last important things." In a letter of January 17, 1980 to Wanja Twan, she wrote:

"When you read this letter, I will be in Arizona to teach a class, then on to San Francisco, to Hawaii—March 19th to St. Pete Florida & Orlando—1st week in April I will be in Atlanta, Georgia to see the dogwood flower festival—May to Israel and Egypt if no war. July to see you all in the Hot Springs and fishing with Peter & his friends—So you see I have a busy schedule but Happy and Well."[53]

As Phyllis Furumoto writes, Mrs. Takata traveled to the Seattle area toward the end of 1980, where she became ill. She died on December 11, 1980—just a few days before her 80th birthday.

Helen Haberly's book tells us that Mrs. Takata "went into transition without making a formal statement of acknowledgement."[54] Bronwen and Frans Stiene also come to the conclusion: "Hawayo Takata had talked for years of naming a successor/s who would continue in her steps but no one had officially been recognized."[55] However, many of the Masters who were close to Mrs. Takata say there was no doubt that Takata would have selected either her granddaughter Phyllis Furumoto and/or Dr. Barbara Ray as her successor (cf. pg. 84) in her last years. As Paul Mitchell mentioned to me, it was not like Mrs. Takata to make official announcements. He read a letter that she wrote to Phyllis Furumoto in which Mrs. Takata said to her granddaughter: "I give it all to you."[56]

The next chapter tells about the course that developed after Mrs. Takata's death. I would like to complete this chapter with Hawayo Takata's own words about the nature of the universe. I think this is a dignified way to close it:

"Here is the great space which surrounds us—the universe. There is endless and enormous energy. It is universal … its ultimate source is the Creator. It can come from the sun or moon or stars. It is a limitless force. It is the source of energy that makes the plants grow, the birds fly. (…) It is Nature. It is God, the power he makes available to his children who seek it."[57]

Acknowledgement

At this point, I would especially like to thank Helen J. Haberly (posthumously), as well as Linda Keiser Mardis of Archedigm Publications who allowed me to use so many quotes from Helen Haberly's book *Reiki: Hawayo Takata's Story*. Furthermore, I would like to expressly thank to Wanja Twan, the author of *In the Light of a Distant Star*, and to Fran Brown, the author of *Living Reiki. Takata's Teachings*, for permitting me to quote from their books. I would especially like to also thank Rolf and Li-Li Holm, as well as Barbara McDaniel from the *Reiki Magazine International* for permission to quote from their numerous articles about Hawayo Takata and her Masters; these articles were a constant source of inspiration for me and offered me many interesting bits of information.

4. Different Paths
The Legacy of Takata

After Mrs. Takata's death, there were several thousand people, primarily in the USA and Canada, who had either been initiated by her into the First and/or Second Degree or by one of the Masters she had initiated. The 22 Masters initiated by Takata were:

George Araki, Dorothy Baba, Ursula Baylow, Rick Bockner, Barbara Brown, Fran Brown, Patricia Ewing, Phyllis Furumoto (Takata's granddaughter), Beth Gray, John Gray, Iris Ishikura, Harry Kuboi, Ethel Lombardi, Barbara McCullough, Mary McFadyen, Paul Mitchell, Bethel Paigh, Shinobu Saito, Virginia Samdahl, Barbara Weber Ray, Wanja Twan, and Kay Yamashita (one of Takata's sisters).[1]

In an interview published in the *Reiki Magazine International,* John Gray talks about the time directly after Takata's death:

"When Takata died in 1980, there were twenty-two of us Masters. One year later, seventeen of us met in the Hawaiian Islands for a week. We talked about Reiki, about the symbols, and gave Reiki treatments. At that time, we acknowledged that Takata's granddaughter, Phyllis Furumoto, was the leader of the Reiki movement. That felt good. I became a member of The Reiki Alliance very soon after it was formed. I have been a member these many years, but in 1999, it was the first time I visited the conference."[2]

All 22 of the Masters initiated by Takata had been invited by Phyllis Furumoto to attend the meeting, which took place in spring of 1982 on the Hawaiian Islands.[3] However, just 17 of them came.

Paul Mitchell remembers the following participants: George Araki, Dorothy Baba, Rick Bockner, Barbara Brown, Fran Brown, Phyllis Furumoto, Beth Gray, John Gray, Ethel Lombardi, Mary McFadyen, Bethel Paigh, Shinobu Saito, Virginia Samdahl, and himself. The majority of those present acknowledged Phyllis Furumoto as the successor of Hawayo Takata.[4]

The Reiki Alliance

At the following meeting, which took place in 1983 in Canada at the home of Barbara Brown[5], The Reiki Alliance, "an alliance of Reiki Masters" with the purpose of supporting each other as teachers in the Usui System was founded.[6] The members of The Reiki Alliance, which currently includes about 600 Reiki Masters throughout the world, acknowledge Phyllis Furumoto as the Grand Master and Lineage Bearer "in the direct spiritual lineage of Mikao Usui, Chujiro Hayashi, and Hawayo Takata."[7]

At the founding of The Reiki Alliance, nine of the Masters initiated by Takata were present: George Araki, Ursula Baylow, Rick Bockner, Barbara Brown, Phyllis Furumoto, Paul Mitchell, Bethel Paigh, Shinobu Saito, and Wanja Twan. Furthermore, other students of Takata and Phyllis Furumoto were there.[8] According to the reports, at least three more Masters initiated by Takata joined soon after it had been established: John Gray, Fran Brown, and Virginia Samdahl.[9] This means that at least 12 of the 22 Masters initiated by Takata were members of The Reiki Alliance during the first years.

Today, The Reiki Alliance sees itself as an organization for Reiki Masters who orientate themselves upon the *Usui Shiki Ryoho* System of Reiki in their practice and teachings (see pgs. 92 ff.). However, as Phyllis Furumoto emphasized in an interview in 2001, "The Reiki Alliance is not the only place where masters of this system, *Usui Shiki Ryoho,* reside. Joining the organization is a choice made by some masters to work together within a community (...) Within the community of the Alliance, masters are consistently confronted with being part of a group, not the leader of the group. It is a challenge and not a validation. I support the nature of this community."[10]

While the Masters initiated by Takata who saw Phyllis Furumoto in the leadership role referred to her as the Grand Master during the early times, she is now primarily seen as the Lineage Bearer within the *Usui Shiki Ryoho*.[11] Mary McFadyen wrote the following about the term "Grand Master" and the assumption that Mrs. Takata called herself "The Grand Master of Reiki":

"It is my understanding that neither Dr. Hayashi nor Mrs. Takata ever referred to themselves as a Grand Master. This form of address was originally used by one of Mrs. Takata's Masters in 1978, when she introduced Mrs. Takata as 'The Grand Master of Reiki' to a group of students who were assembled to take a Reiki course. The title continued to be used by Mrs. Takata's Masters as a demonstration of honor and respect for her."[12]

The Reiki Association

In addition to The Reiki Alliance, there was a second organization that developed out of the work of the Masters and students who were initiated by Hawayo Takata. This was The Reiki Association, which was founded during Takata's lifetime (cf. pgs. 96 ff.). This organization also continues to exist today; however, it has been renamed a number of times and is now called The Radiance Technique International Association, Inc. (TRTIA).[13]

TRTIA is now an internationally oriented, non-profit association that works for the worldwide dissemination of The Radiance Technique®, among other things (see pg. 96). Anyone who would like to support this and other goals of the association can become a member. In addition, there are national associations in various countries that work closely with the international association.

In the early 1980s, there were Masters initiated by Takata who were members in both organizations, The Reiki Alliance and The Reiki Association. For example, Fran Brown writes that Mrs. Takata had asked her to work with and support both Phyllis Furumoto and Dr. Barbara Ray. At that time, Fran Brown was a member of both organizations.[14] Virginia Samdahl, who had initiated Dr. Barbara Ray into the First and Second Degree, was also initially a member in both organizations, report Bronwen and Frans Stiene.[15] Fran Brown writes the following on this topic:

"I guess Takata made Phyllis a Master about the same time she initiated Barbara. When she talked to me about these things, she had great faith in the spirituality of Barbara. And she knew that Barbara had the know-how to make an organization go. She had hoped that they would work together. Phyllis would bring the Oriental side out and Barbara would do the organizing—that was her idea at the time. But they could not work together; Barbara would have none of that. She wanted the whole wad and she was going to take it to heights never dreamed of. And so all I did there (at The Reiki Association, author's note) was receive Barbara's newsletter, until they stopped sending it."[16]

Dr. Barbara Ray was among the five Masters initiated by Takata who did not come to the meeting in spring of 1982 on the Hawaiian Islands. As Phyllis Furumoto wrote in the *Reiki Magazine International,* after this meeting in which the majority of the Masters attending had recognized her as Takata's successor, she attempted to speak with Barbara Ray about it. According to Phyllis, she already knew at this time that Barbara Ray considered herself to be the person who Takata had prepared to be her successor.[17] As she writes, Phyllis wanted to make her an offer to work together since she was convinced that Barbara Ray could give people something that she, Phyllis, could not give them and vice versa. However, as Phyllis writes, Barbara Ray was not open to working together, which led to the end of their relationship.[18]

As far as I know, a description of this meeting on the part of Dr. Barbara Ray, as well as her reasons for not participating in the meeting on the Hawaiian Islands, has not been published anywhere up to now. Although I offered an interview in the *Reiki Magazin* to Dr. Barbara Ray on several occasions in recent years, she was unfortunately not interested, according to statements by Ulrike Wolf, the author of the book *Die Radiance Technik,* who was gracious enough to pass on my inquiries to Dr. Ray.

When Phyllis Furumoto told the Reiki history in its legendary form at the German-language 2002 Reiki Festival in Gersfeld, she also spoke for the first time about the period around Takata's death. She disclosed how she visited her grandmother in the hospital and how Takata had asked her to go the very next day to a Reiki seminar that had already been planned for a long time and that she, Takata, was actually scheduled to hold. She asked Phyllis to take her place there since there were still many people waiting to learn Reiki.[19]

"Leiki"

As Bronwen and Frans Stiene describe it, Alice Takata Furumoto, the daughter of Hawayo Takata and the mother of Phyllis Furumoto, put together a little booklet in 1982 that is also called *The Gray Book,* which she gave to the Masters initiated by Takata.[20] The booklet with the title of *Leiki* contains writings by Hawayo Takata that include the topics of the First and Second Degree, treatments, hand positions for specific complaints, principles, nutrition, a copy of Hawayo Takata's Reiki certificate that was filled out by Dr. Hayashi, a list of the Masters initiated by Takata, photos of

Hawayo Takata, and the "Treatment Plan" (cf. pg. 160) written by Dr. Hayashi in Japanese characters.[21] The title of the booklet, *Leiki*, was probably selected because it refers to the Japanese pronunciation of the word "Reiki," which is somewhere between the "L" and the "R" in terms of the beginning letter. Bronwen and Frans Stiene write the following about it:

"The Japanese language has no correlation with English or its pronunciations. The *kanji* for 'rei' is officially spelt with an 'R' when translating into English and is therefore pronounced with an 'R' (even though the Japanese pronunciation might sound similar to what is understood as an 'L' in English)."[22]

At the end of my training period for becoming a Reiki Master, in November 2000 in Idaho, I had the opportunity to hold a copy of *The Gray Book* in my hands. In addition to the above-mentioned contents, I also found that it had a formulation of the Principles in Old English that goes back to Hawayo Takata and is reproduced on pg. 67 of this book.

Worldwide Dissemination

In the 1980s, the worldwide dissemination of the Usui System in the form created by Dr. Hayashi and Mrs. Takata increased rapidly because of the 22 Masters initiated by Takata. As Mary McFadyen writes:

"Until the death of Mrs. Takata Reiki was known in Japan, the United States, and Canada. This changed dramatically the following year. At that time I was invited to teach Reiki in Europe by Brigitte Müller, who later became the first German Reiki Master. In the summer of 1981 I taught Reiki I courses in Hamburg and Frankfurt in Germany and at the Findhorn Community in Scotland. This began the incredibly rapid spread of Reiki worldwide, which still continues today. At the present time I believe that quite possibly there is no country in the world which does not have someone who has the healing energy of Reiki."[23]

In addition to the USA and Canada, the countries in which a great many people have learned the Usui System of Reiki up to now primarily include—as far as I know—Germany, Austria, Holland, Great Britain, France, Brazil, Russia, India, and Australia. The Usui System of Reiki has recently also become more popular in Japan (cf. pg. 163). We can assume that there are at least some Reiki Teachers and practitioners in almost every country of the earth by now.

Takata's Masters

The Masters initiated by Takata, as well as the Masters initiated by Phyllis Furumoto and other Masters initiated in the lineage of Takata, were those through whom the Usui System of Reiki has spread throughout the world. I have personally become acquainted with some of Masters initiated by Takata during the course of recent years. One of these Masters ultimately became my teacher: Paul Mitchell.

In the spring of 1996, I participated in an Aikido workshop offered by Paul at the *Reiki Mandala Center* in the Lüneburg Heath, Germany. Paul holds this workshop only for Reiki practitioners, and it focuses more on the aspect of self-realization than martial arts. During the first days, Paul frequently had me come to the front during the exercise periods to demonstrate something using me as an example. I noticed that I could learn a lot from him and felt drawn to him. A few days later, as I sat next to Paul during the group dinner, I had the inspiration to ask if he would accept me as one of his students. However, I first asked whether he would have some time right after dinner because there was something I wanted to ask him. We made an appointment for half an hour later in his room. The following half hour was a very long one. When it had finally passed, I went directly to Paul's room, knocked on the door, was invited in, sat down, and directly asked him whether he would accept me as a student. He had obviously already had a premonition about what I had in mind, and I was more than happy to receive a "yes" in response to my question.

During my training period, I traveled to see Paul on a regular basis whenever he held Reiki seminars in Germany—this was usually in Bad Sobernheim, a small town near the city of Mainz. I was a guest in Paul's seminars during these visits and learned simply by absorbing the situations, as well as giving and receiving Reiki. In addition, I had individual conversations with Paul and gave him Reiki treatments. We walked together through the city, ran errands, and sat in the sidewalk cafés and drank cappuccino.

In the course of that year, I attended additional Aikido seminars offered by Paul in Germany and the USA, participated in large events with him and Phyllis Furumoto. When I received my initiation into the Master Degree in November of 2000, this marked the end of my five-year training period, as well as the start of a new phase with Reiki as a beginning Reiki Master.

I am pleased to have Paul's support for this book and that he has contributed a practical exercise. The exercise for the first Principle, "Just for today, do not anger," on page 89 stems from Paul's seminars on researching the Reiki Principles. It can help us deal with the topic of anger.

Encounters

In addition to Paul Mitchell, I have also become more closely acquainted with Phyllis Furumoto over time, although a closer

Exploring my Anger
By Paul Mitchell

Do this alone or with a partner. Take a sheet of paper and write at the top: "I get angry when…"

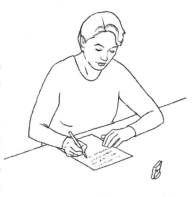

Exploring

If you are working with a partner, they will hold the paper and write down what you say. They will begin the sentence: "I get angry when…" and you will complete the sentence, saying whatever comes to your mind. After they have written what you said, they will begin the sentence again and you will respond. It is important to do this for five to seven minutes without stopping. Whatever comes to your mind, allow yourself to say it. If you are doing it alone, set a timer and do the process yourself without stopping.

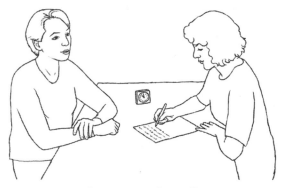

"I get angry when …"

When you are done, read through your statements. Notice which ones are most personal.

I learned many years ago that the most common causes of anger are when our ego is threatened and when we don't get what we want. Think about this. Then consider this question: What is underneath your anger? Be specific. You will most likely find that anger is usually a secondary response. Find out what your first feeling is and have the courage to stay with it. As you do this, you will become angry much less.

contact between us has actually only been established since the evening of my Master initiation. Together with other guests, I was invited to her house and after dinner we played music together. I experience Phyllis as a very clear woman who lives her truth— simply and directly. And I notice how I lack the words to describe the depths that I perceive in her and cannot express.

I became closely acquainted with three other Masters initiated by Takata at the annual conference of The Reiki Alliance in 2002 in Germany: Rick Bockner, Shinobu Saito, and Wanja Twan. I experienced my encounters with Wanja Twan as especially impressive. She once sat directly next to me during a lecture and I felt the unbelievable energetic presence that radiated from her. During a moment when she slightly raised her arm and moved it back and forth, I felt how much Reiki radiated from her just through this movement.

A few days later, Wanja gave the so-called "Reiki Blessings" in a separate room. I also wanted to receive this type of "blessing," which Wanja says she learned from Mrs. Takata. So I got into the long line of those waiting admission to Wanja and her daughter Kristina, with whom she gave the "blessings." The crowd was so large that I could not get in on that day, but it did work out on the next day. The "blessing" turned out to be an energy transmission. I spontaneously felt myself being lifted up energetically. Shortly afterward, Wanja said something like: "Green grass, you should walk on green grass." In response to my question as to what she meant by that, she said that she felt it would be good for me to walk barefoot through meadows or on sand in order to feel a direct connection to the earth. I was totally perplexed, but felt that she was right.

In the following months, whenever I went through a park I simply took off my shoes and socks and walked barefoot on the grass—and it felt good. I later bought myself sandals for the summer months.

And now in the summer, whenever the weather is warm enough, I am happy that I do not need to wear socks and outdoor shoes anymore.

The "Reiki Blessing" that I received from Wanja reminds me of the "Reiju energy transmissions" that I had received from Don Alexander (cf. pg. 25). We can assume that both have the same origin, which probably goes back to Mikao Usui.

Transition

More than one-third of the 22 Masters initiated by Takata are already no longer alive today. Some passed away just a few years after Takata's death. Up to the year 2004, eight of the 22 Masters initiated by Takata died: Dorothy Baba († about 1983), Iris Ishikura († 1984), Bethel Phaigh († on January 3, 1986), Kay Yamashita († in May of 1987), Barbara McCullough († in the late 1980s), Ursula Baylow († mid-1990s), Virginia Samdahl († 1994), and Barbara Brown († on Easter Sunday of 2000).[24]

Developments

While most of the Masters initiated by Takata joined and/or helped found The Reiki Alliance during the 1980s and Dr. Barbara Ray continued Takata's work with The Reiki Association in her own way (cf. pgs. 96–97), some of the other Masters initiated by Takata took highly individual paths. For example, Ethel Lombardi, who was already initiated as a Master in 1976, reportedly developed her own system of laying-on hands in the time after Takata's death: Mari-EL, which is based on the Usui System of Reiki.[25]

Furthermore, Harry M. Kuboi, who was the sixth of the Masters initiated by Takata, developed very individualistic views of Reiki over time. As Bronwen and Frans Stiene write, he is now convinced that the majority of people initiated into Reiki have "negative Reiki," which is why he no longer teaches the Usui System. Instead, he does energetic cleansings for people who have been initiated into Reiki and desire this.[26]

In addition, Iris Ishikura, the tenth of the Masters initiated by Takata, reportedly has developed a new Reiki system on the basis of the Usui System together with Arthur Robertson, an earlier student of Virginia Samdahl[27]. This system is called *Raku Kei Reiki* and integrates Tibetan symbols, among other things. This new system of Reiki has consequently inspired many more forms such as *Tera Mai Reiki, Johrei Reiki, and Karuna Reiki®*.[28] Mrs. Takata supposedly told her Master student Iris Ishikura to initiate only a total of three people into the Master Degree. Iris Ishikura only initiated her daughter and Arthur Robertson into the Master Degree before she died in 1984.[29]

Usui Shiki Ryoho

In the late 1980s, with the increasing worldwide spread of the Usui System, a development started that created an abundance of new forms and ways of working with the universal life energy of Reiki. These were generally based on the Usui System. However, as Paul Mitchell has discovered, it was not always clear when changes were made in respect to the form taught by Takata.[30] In an interview, Paul Mitchell made the following comments:

"At a conference of The Reiki Alliance in 1992, Phyllis was asked to define The Usui System. This question came as a result of the situation that different forms of Reiki were proliferating, and everyone was calling what they did by the same name. The masters at this conference believed they were within a certain system that was practiced and passed on, but because of the difference of forms and interpretations, there was growing confusion about what that was exactly. Phyllis and I took on the project of answering these questions. We did this by exploring our own memories of what Mrs. Takata carried and taught, as well as consulting with other masters that Mrs. Takata had trained. We also sat with circles of masters exploring this question. Some time in the next year, Phyllis awoke one morning, went to her computer, and wrote an article for her newsletter in which she named the four aspects and nine elements of the practice *Usui Shiki Ryoho*. It is important to know that when we read them, the response was: 'Yes, this is my experience of what I received and practice.' Our task was to find the language to describe what we had received from Mrs. Takata, not to make something up. For the past ten years now we have lived with these elements and find that they still do, in fact, describe the system as it was passed down to us."[31]

The four aspects and nine elements of the *Usui Shiki Ryoho* System that resulted from this process summarize what Phyllis Furumoto, Paul Mitchell, and other Masters initiated by Takata see as the core of their teachings.[32] In the words of Phyllis Furumoto, the four aspects of *Usui Shiki Ryoho* are "Healing, Personal Growth, Spiritual Discipline, and Mystic Order. These aspects revolve and radiate out from a central core of practice and philosophy that will be called the form. There are nine tenants of the form: Initiations, Symbols, Treatments, Oral Tradition, History, Form of Teaching, Precepts, Lineage, and Money."[33]

As Paul Mitchell states, "*Usui Shiki Ryoho* is the Japanese name for the System of Reiki that came to the Western world through Hawaii in 1938. It was taught in Hawaii first by Dr. Hayashi with Mrs. Takata and then he entrusted the practice to her. In the notarized certificate that Dr. Hayashi prepared for Mrs. Takata, the practice she received is described in several ways: The Usui System of Reiki Healing, The Usui System of Drugless Healing, and Dr. Usui's Reiki

System of Healing. The words *Usui Shiki Ryoho* translate in English to The Usui System (or method) of Healing."[34]

In 1993, Phyllis Furumoto created the Office of the Grandmaster (OGM) of *Usui Shiki Ryoho* together with Paul Mitchell. While Phyllis Furumoto, as the successor of Hawayo Takata, understands herself to be the Lineage Bearer of *Usui Shiki Ryoho,* Paul Mitchell works next to her as the Head of the Discipline of *Usui Shiki Ryoho.* Together, the two of them mutually embody the Office of the Grandmaster of *Usui Shiki Ryoho.* The process that led to this development is described in the following by Paul Mitchell:

"From our first meeting, Phyllis and I experienced a strong connection. After her grandmother died in 1980, I was one of the masters who responded to Phyllis' call to be part of a master community and was one of the founding members of The Reiki Alliance. Very early on, in 1984, Phyllis asked me to work with her in the training and preparation of the masters she was training and initiating. I supported her in her role of Lineage Bearer, and she delegated some responsibilities to me. In 1989 there were some personal problems in our relationship, and I stopped working with her. In 1992 it became clear to me that this personal separation was not serving the Reiki community. As I looked beyond the personal, I felt called to share with Phyllis somehow in the role of Grand Master, to carry and care for the system and its integrity. We arranged a meeting. It was one of those magical healing moments where all the past stuff just fell away, and we were present to one another. I shared with her my perception of my role, and she acknowledged that it was also true for her. The first recognition came from her, which seemed essential and right."[35]

"One of the energetic components of the Office of the Grandmaster," according to Paul Mitchell, "is to just hold the energy of the system as a still point for the Reiki community."[36]

Form and Practice

The *Usui Shiki Ryoho* System of Reiki consists of three degrees or levels: the First Degree, the Second Degree, and the Master Level. Within the scope of a First Degree seminar there are four initiations. The participants learn the hand positions for self-treatment, as well as for the treatment of other people, and are familiarized with the Principles and History of the Usui System. Within the scope of a Second Degree seminar, which should be taken six months after the First Degree seminar at the earliest, three symbols are taught. With the associated initiation, the participants receive the abilities to intensify the Reiki energy, to do mental healing, and to do distant healing. For the Master Degree, a longer training period is required. This can mean several years while the students enter into a deeper relationship with the initiating Master. After the conclusion of the Master training, the students themselves are Masters and can initiate others into the First and Second Degree. Masters of *Usui Shiki Ryoho* are expected to wait about ten years before they in turn initiate others into the Master Degree, in case they even consider this as their task.

Practicing *Usui Shiki Ryoho* on a regular basis consists of daily self-treatment with Reiki and the sincere effort to translate the contents of the Principles into actions in everyday life.[37] The common form of the Principles within the *Usui Shiki Ryoho* is now:

> "Just for today, do not anger.
> Just for today, do not worry.
> Honor your parents, teachers, and elders.
> Earn your living honestly.
> Show gratitude to every living thing."[38]

In the *Usui Shiki Ryoho* System of Reiki, the practitioners find a simple form of the Usui System that dates back to Dr. Hayashi and Mrs. Takata. This system is now taught by thousands of Reiki Masters throughout the world. At the same time, it depicts the basic form of what has spread internationally as the "Usui System of Reiki" during the past 25 years. As a result, this form of the Usui System can be considered the starting point for the worldwide dissemination of the Usui System, as well as the basic form for all other systems that have arisen from it.

⌒

The Radiance Technique®

In 1983, some years after Takata's death, Dr. Barbara Ray published the book *The Reiki Factor*.[39] This was the first book about Reiki in the Western world. In it, she wrote about "this science of Transcendental energy"[40], just as she had received it from Mrs. Takata. According to her, Dr. Barbara Ray received from Takata "the Keys to this Transcendental, Cosmic energy science in its entirety in order to keep the continuity of making this precious science in a new cycle and in a new context and to continue to protect, maintain and preserve this unique science whole and intact."[41]

Dr. Barbara Ray is still the head of The Reiki Association, which was established in 1980 and now bears the name The Radiance Technique International Association, Inc. (TRTIA) (cf. pg. 83). Among other things, the internationally oriented organization works toward the worldwide dissemination of *The Radiance Technique®*. This is now the main term used for the system that Dr. Ray claims to have received from Mrs. Takata and which she and the teachers belonging to TRTIA teach.

Since Mrs. Takata's death, according to Dr. Ray, "extensive fragmentation, misrepresentation, confusion in thinking and lack of correct information and knowledge have occured concerning the polluted, disconnected and partial 'something called reiki' which is not at all the actual intact science that was rediscovered and passed on by Dr. Usui."[42]

For this reason, according to Dr. Barbara Ray in her text "Historical Perspectives on The Radiance Technique®, Authentic Reiki®, Real Reiki®, TRT®", published on the website of TRTIA, "The Radiance Technique®, Authentic Reiki® and Real Reiki® are the main terms registered now in the necessity of denoting and distinguishing, from 'whatever reiki things', the intact and complete Cosmic energy science rediscovered by Dr. Usui."[43]

The disapproving attitude on the part of Dr. Barbara Ray and the teachers who I know from the TRTIA toward anyone who practices and teaches other forms of the Usui System makes it difficult for me to write about *The Radiance Technique®*. In an article about *The Radiance Technique®* written by Frank Doerr, author and Reiki Master in the tradition of *Usui Shiki Ryoho* and *Usui-Do* for the German-language *Reiki Magazin* (because none of the teachers who teach *The Radiance Technique®* wanted to write such an article for a Reiki magazine), he says:

"An essential characteristic of The Radiance Technique® is the system of seven degrees. The First and Second Degrees appear to correspond with the learning contents of these degrees in the current Western Reiki styles. In the higher degrees, there are additional subdivisions into an A and B lineage, whereby the A Degree serves personal growth and transformation while the B Degree contains an additional attunement and teaching capabilities. In my opinion, this is where the origin of the subdivision of the classical Master Degree into the Master and the Teacher's Degree has been assumed by large portions of the independent Reiki scene. However, The Radiance Technique® makes a stronger differentiation: In lll B, students learn to give Degrees l and ll; in V B, they learn to teach lll, and with the Vll B they can teach all of the degrees."[44]

Seven Degrees?

In contrast to all of the other traditional forms of the Usui System, which usually include three degrees, *The Radiance Technique®* always speaks of seven degrees. These circumstances have already led to numerous assumptions of various types in the past. For example, many practitioners of *The Radiance Technique®* apparently believe that Phyllis Furumoto just received an incomplete version of the Usui System from her grandmother. This assumption is contradicted by the fact that, as far as I know, actually all of the Masters initiated by Takata, with the exception of Dr. Barbara Ray, teach or taught a System with three degrees. However, Dr. Barbara Ray considers herself the only Master who received the complete system from Mrs. Takata. Yet, the question arises why she did not bring this System into the community of Takata's Masters (cf. pg. 84).

Furthermore, the first English edition of the book *The Reiki Factor* by Dr. Barbara Ray, which was published in the USA by Exposition Press in 1983, only speaks of three Reiki Degrees; however, Dr. Ray later wrote about seven degrees in further editions of this same work. From my perspective, this does not necessarily support the assumption that the system actually includes seven degrees.[45]

Another point that speaks against an original system with seven degrees is the fact that all of the information available up to now about the beginnings of the system from the time of Mikao Usui also speak of three degrees and make absolutely no mention of seven degrees (cf. Chapter 1 and 2). Moreover, it is conspicuous that the information published in recent years about the origins of the Usui System have barely been noticed—or not at all—by many practitioners of *The Radiance Technique®*. This is my impression. For example, the 2004 German-language book *Die Radiance Technik* by Ulrike Wolf states that the history of *The Radiance Technique®* has remained unbroken for about 150 years up to now and that *The*

Radiance Technique® was rediscovered in the middle of the 19th Century by Dr. Mikao Usui.[46] (As we have known for some time now, Mikao Usui was not even born until 1865. All of the existing sources assume that he began no earlier than 1910 in developing the Reiki method of healing called *Reiki Ryoho.)*

The Course of Things

What unites many of the Masters initiated by Takata is a long-held mistrust against the further developments of the Usui System that have occurred since the mid-1980s in the course of the system spreading throughout the world. For a long time, many people responded like Barbara Brown, who describes her own process in relation to this occurrence:

"I had nothing to worry about. I was never angry. At least, I thought I was not. Until the change in Reiki when people started teaching it differently than Takata, and then I suddenly began to feel resentment toward them. A feeling that they should not be doing this and how dare they change it. I did not recognize it as an anger, I thought it was just criticism of people who did not really trust or respect Takata and her teaching. All Reiki in America came from Takata, therefore if there was any difference, it came through other people changing it. How can a newcomer in a western country hear about Reiki and say 'I know better'? To me it was astonishing. I myself knew that I did not know better. I could not possibly know better. I had not spent the time at it."[47]

As Barbara Brown continues to tell the story, she managed to change her attitude about this with time. When she was finally able to let go completely of her anger, she was spontaneously filled with light and joy.[48]

Five years later, in the spring of 2004, Paul Mitchell summarized his process with the changes in the Usui System according to Hawayo Takata as follows:

"Over the years, my feelings and reactions to the changes and interpretations of the practice of Reiki have progressed. First there was a disbelief, sadness, outrage, and judgment, a feeling that my practice was more pure and better than others. Then I moved on to resignation, acceptance, tolerance, understanding, sometimes even compassion. I have not forgotten any of the steps to this dance. I can still do them all, depending on how centered I am in any given moment."[49]

In the further course of the article, he concludes: "Where do I truly want to put my energy? The answer is simple: acceptance, tolerance, understanding, and compassion. The practice, however, can be difficult."[50]

Many Reiki practitioners who have learned one of the currently abundant forms and expressions of the Usui System may find the process that many of the Masters initiated by Takata obviously went through to be quite strange—especially in view of the currently well-known fact that even the form of the Usui System taught by Takata was already a further development of the form originally developed by Mikao Usui. However, we should not forget that this was not a well-known fact in the 1970s and 1980s in the USA. And that Mrs. Takata, in contrast to many others who have often made changes in the system shortly after their initiation into the Master Degree, could look back on almost 40 years of practicing the system before she passed it on in a different form.

The proper balance between maintaining traditional elements and the further development of these elements or the addition of new elements is certainly an important topic for every Reiki Teacher.

Those who want to experience continuing authentic spiritual and personal development cannot avoid it.

The following chapter will introduce some of the new directions and styles based on the Usui System of Reiki that have arisen since the 1990s and have attained a certain extent of validity since then.

5. The Variety
New Directions and Styles

In the course of the years, various new styles, directions, and systems have developed from the Usui System of Reiki. This chapter offers a representative selection of them.

New Systems

"For some 20 years now, new systems of energy work on the basis of *Usui Shiki Ryoho* (Usui System of Natural Healing) created by Dr. Mikao Usui have emerged in the Western world. In Japan, this development already began at the latest after Dr. Usui's death in 1926 by some of his students according to their own ideas. (…) So it is not a new development that the form of the Usui System of Reiki has changed, been expanded, and is used in different ways. People generally try to make the best of their situation—and this also includes adapting what they have learned to their own personal circumstances and their individual type of philosophy in order to better take care of themselves and those around them."[1]

These are the words with which Walter Lübeck began his article on *Rainbow Reiki,* which he founded, in the German-language *Reiki Magazin.* In the further course of the text, he points out that even the Usui System of Natural Healing developed in keeping with this description because Mikao Usui spent decades studying and trying out a great variety of spiritual paths in Japan and other countries. He ultimately adapted what he learned to his view of the world, as well the people around him and their needs at that time.[2]

Rainbow Reiki

Walter Lübeck learned all three degrees of *Usui Shiki Ryoho* in the late 1980s from Brigitte Müller, the first German Reiki Master.[3] Already during this time, he formed the foundation for the later form of *Rainbow Reiki,* which he officially called into being in 1994.[4] In an article about Walter Lübeck, Sylvia-Manuela Regler wrote:

"During his training to become a Reiki Master, he was expected to largely remember all of the teaching contents without writing them down. However, Walter Lübeck wanted to 'take along' as much as possible for himself and his subsequent teaching activities and therefore took notes anyway. At the same time that he was training to become a Reiki Master, he also became intensively involved with the Huna teachings, as well as working with his 'Higher Self,' 'Inner Child,' and shamanism. This is something that was not at all commonplace in the Reiki scene of that time. Later, he began to integrate further methods, such as the use of healing stones, Zen meditation, and Feng Shui into his Reiki work and trainings."[5]

In the following section, Walter Lübeck explains the *Rainbow Reiki* that he developed in a brief succinct way:

"Rainbow Reiki was created in the late 1980s and early '90s. The foundation on which it started to develop at that time was traditional Reiki of the Western variety as transmitted by Hawayo Takata. Traditional Japanese methods were integrated into it. Research into the roots of the 'Usui System of Natural Healing with Reiki' provided the approaches of Dr. Mikao Usui and Dr. Chujiro Hayashi. This includes the underlying spiritual wisdom such as the mystic healing practices of the Buddha Dainichi Nyorai. Together with the traditional initiation rituals, the four symbols, their Mantras and the fundamental techniques of Reiki

103

energy work these now form the basis of Rainbow Reiki. Our own developments such as the essences technique, the cooperation with the Inner Child, the Higher Self and the angels, KarmaClearing and systematic chakra work came about in the course of the years. We sought continuously to facilitate healing in areas where it had not been possible to work with traditional Reiki, or at least not satisfactorily. (...) Just as in Mikao Usui's Reiki schools, meditation has a central place in Rainbow Reiki. (...) Anyone who learns Rainbow Reiki is simultaneously studying traditional Reiki and newly developed spiritual energy work. These additional techniques, initiations, symbols and Mantras have been created as a result of counseling and seminar practice as well as through spiritual research. (...) Rainbow Reiki is taught throughout the world and hundreds of thousands of Reiki enthusiasts have been applying it for many years now."[6]

Unsolved Mystery

About his motivation for creating this new approach based upon the Usui System of Reiki, Walter Lübeck wrote:

"There are still so many unsolved mysteries, and so I don't even want to stop exploring Rainbow Reiki. However, solely the fact that a certain Rainbow Reiki technique works isn't enough for me on its own. Since I like to take responsibility for what I do, it's important for me to comprehend how something functions, exactly what I'm doing, and why it produces certain effects, and under which circumstances something doesn't work."[7]

In this "detective work," as Walter Lübeck calls his research work with a twinkle in his eye, he has found a great deal of support on the part of other Reiki enthusiasts from the very beginning. He has also benefited from the knowledge that came with his naturopathic and psychological training and years of spiritual practice. Many useful perceptions and information were also virtually given to him.[8] He writes: "Today I know that my guardian angel, my Higher Self, and my spiritual teachers, above all the Great Goddess, the mother of us all, have done a great deal to direct my attention to the right things and situations and gradually open me up to certain perceptions."[9]

According to Walter Lübeck, the name "Rainbow Reiki" symbolizes "the harmonious connection of heaven and earth and the openness for everything that helps us take the path to the divine (the colors of the spectrum). In addition, the rainbow has a special personal significance for me since I spent a number of very beautiful lifetimes, which were very important lives for me, on the submerged continent of Lemuria in about 10,000 B.C. Today I apply much of what I was permitted to learn back then while in the service of the Great Goddess in my practice and for myself. Lemuria was also called the 'Land of the Rainbow.'"[10]

Degrees and Advanced Training Opportunities

According to Walter Lübeck, there are "no prerequisites necessary for the First Degree in Rainbow Reiki. For the Second Degree, the precondition is either the First Degree in the traditional Western Usui System or in Rainbow Reiki. Rainbow Reiki seminars on the First and Second Degrees should not be confused with the customary Reiki seminars since—in addition to the authentic traditional contents—they include about 90 percent of original methods, symbols, and mantras that only exist in Rainbow Reiki."[11]

Anyone who wants to use *Rainbow Reiki* "professionally within a counseling or medical practice should attend the seminars for the Rainbow Reiki Practitioner and the Rainbow Reiki Master Practitioner, in addition to the First and Second Degree in Rainbow

Reiki. Upon request, a test can be given afterward and an appropriate certificate (Rainbow Reiki Master Practitioner—Professional Level) can be issued."[12]

"The Rainbow Reiki Master/Teacher training is divided into three complete trainings that build upon each other that last about two years. Every portion contains about 300 instructional hours, as well as diverse materials for home studies and, of course, personal conversations."[13]

According to Walter Lübeck, the very extensive contents of *Rainbow Reiki,* such as those in the Second Degree seminars, can be deepened by the possibility of repeated participation as a guest. This allows each student to glean from the information offered whatever is individually especially useful and interesting. In addition, there are comprehensive written documents for each seminar that explain all of the essentials in precise detail.[14]

Those who have already trained in traditional Reiki according to Hawayo Takata as a Master and have at least two years of experience as a seminar leader can learn to instruct the First and Second Degrees of *Rainbow Reiki* in an abbreviated training, the RR Instructor Training. This includes an emphasis on the knowledge of Rainbow Reiki I and Rainbow Reiki ll, as well as the initiation training related to these seminars.[15]

Projects

I met Walter Lübeck for the first time at the DGH Congress for Spiritual Healing in Göttingen, Germany, in September 2002. Walter participated in the congress as a speaker and had just held a lecture on the topic of "Learning to Feel Subtle Healing Energies." Jürgen Kindler and I were also participating in the congress as speakers, including a lecture on the topic of "What

Comes after the Reiki Master Degree?" During the lunch break, we used the opportunity to sit down with Walter and talk about possible mutual projects such as the production of a special edition of the *Reiki Magazin* in cooperation with *Windpferd Verlag*, which publishes Walter's numerous books in German, as well as organizing a nation-wide German Reiki Symposium in the near future. We had a stimulating conversation and translated some of our ideas into action in the following period of time. I have repeatedly experienced the work with Walter to be inspiring, as well as pragmatic and solution-oriented, which is very advantageous in its concrete realization.

In spring of 2004, Walter opened the first German Reiki Clinic in Aerzen, near Hanover. This is also the home of the *Reiki-Do Institut* that he runs, which is recognized as a training institute by the DGH, the German umbrella organization for spiritual healing. Some of Walter's many books and publications on Reiki and other spiritual topics have been translated into 15 languages. The exercise on page 108 comes from his book *Rainbow Reiki.*[16] Walter describes it as follows:

"I came across the Reiki powerball technique while searching for a more simple, intensive, yet still gentle method of chakra work that can also reach and harmonize the deeper levels of an energy center. Other methods have a hard time going beyond the relatively superficial areas of a chakra in their effects and temporarily create a fair amount of disorder in the process or they can only be successfully applied by people who have a great deal of experience. The Reiki powerball technique has proved itself to be quite successful up to now. Even extensive blocks are usually not an obstacle for it."[17]

Chakra Development with the Reiki Powerball
By Walter Lübeck

Step 1: Creating the Reiki Powerball

Before the powerball can develop its effect on other people and objects, you must first create it.

To do this, hold your hands, palms facing each other, about 20 to 30 centimeters (8 to 12 inches) apart at the level of your heart and about 30 centimeters (12 inches) from your body. Wait a moment and feel your way into the energy that increasingly collects between your hands. Now gently move them back and forth, like grass swaying in the wind. Change the distance between them somewhat while you do this. First in one direction, then the other. Feel how the power continues to grow. Feel the resistance of the Reiki powerball when you move your hands a bit closer to each other. Perceive how your hands are gently held back by the energy when you slowly pull them away from each other. During the entire exercise, be sure that the palms of your hands always remain facing each other, that they don't touch each other, but also that there is no more than a distance of more than 40 centimeters (16 inches) between them.

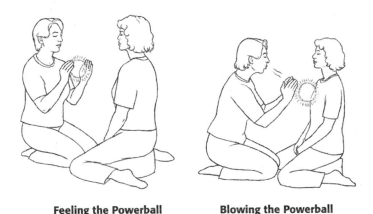

Feeling the Powerball   **Blowing the Powerball**

Step 2: Application of the Reiki Powerball

Continue to hold your hands with the insides turned towards each other, about 20 to 30 centimeters (8 to 12 inches) apart from each other. In this position, move them to a distance of about 30 centimeters

(12 inches) from each other in front of one of your exercise partner's six lower major chakras (you should only work with the seventh chakra, the crown energy center, when you have had enough experience in dealing with energy work in general and this exercise in particular).

Now blow gently and constantly through your hands to the corresponding chakra until you have exhaled completely. Repeat this process—the blowing—at least two more times. If you haven't had much experience with this exercise and/or the way your exercise partner reacts to it, then don't blow more than six or seven times. While doing this, direct your attention to the energy that you move through the power of your breath and the effect it has in the chakra to which you are directing it. After each time you blow the energy into the chakra, ask your partner about his perceptions. If some sort of strong imbalance becomes perceptible and doesn't disappear on its own after a few minutes, help him ground himself by treating the upper area of the soles of his feet for several minutes. In difficult cases, alternate provide the foot soles and the navel area directly with Reiki and have your partner breathe into the hara. This is a switching point for vital energy, not a chakra, found about two fingers beneath the navel on the central line of the body.

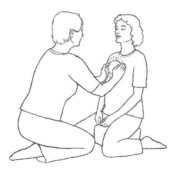

Moving the Powerball

Another variation of this exercise consists of moving the Reiki powerball slowly and as close as possible to exercise partner's corresponding chakra by guiding your hands in this direction. During the first attempts with this method, don't establish the contact for more than about 30 seconds. Ask your partner to keep you informed about his perceptions. If necessary, ground him.

Please note: If you move your hands apart at some point, in order to do something else with them, for example, to treat your client's feet or do chakra balancing, you have to recreate the Reiki powerball each time before you can work with it again!

The effect of this exercise: A large amount of concentrated Reiki energy collects between your hands as a result of this exercise. The breath has a special quality that strongly supports the impact and reception of subtle energies in the human energy system, particularly in the chakras. The chakra provided with Reiki in this manner can more easily free itself of blocks that impede its natural function and more quickly balance a possible charging deficit or release an excess of energy. Most people feel refreshed, strengthened, centered, and more relaxed after a treatment with the Reiki powerball.

Laws and Philosophy

In his book *Rainbow Reiki*, Walter Lübeck devotes several pages to the laws of the system that he has founded. Here are some excerpts from it:

"1. Reiki is a non-polar force. It is neither yin nor yang. Both hands of a person initiated traditionally into Reiki automatically transmit the same vibration—Reiki, to be precise. (…).

2. Reiki supports the living processes in everything with which it comes in contact. To the extent that this is permitted, Reiki is drawn in and influences the development of liveliness in a certain physical or mental, emotional, and spiritual area. (…)

3. Reiki isn't a form of energy capable of directly filling out material or energetic deficits or reducing energetic excesses.

4. Reiki is drawn in by the Inner Child/body consciousness of the recipient. (…)

5. The extent to which Reiki is drawn in depends on how much the Inner Child of the Reiki recipient trusts the practitioner, the situation, and the purpose of developing a new form of behavior triggered by Reiki, a new physical and mental, emotional, and spiritual state, as well as his general need for animating impulses. (…)"[18]

Rainbow Reiki, according to Walter Lübeck, also has "an extensive philosophical background based upon the contents taught by Dr. Mikao Usui such as the five Principles. In addition, it uses the three maxims: 'strengthening individual responsibility,' 'promotion of the ability to love,' and 'expanding the consciousness.' This and other components of the Rainbow Reiki philosophy help students learn to think in a spiritual, and therefore healthy and natural way. (…) The Rainbow Reiki philosophy helps people

111

understand life from the divine perspective, find peace within themselves, with fellow human beings, and with the world, and recognizes the individually appropriate path to the light and to love. We should not equate understanding with healing and development. However, long-term, individually responsible healing and spiritual development are frequently only possible on the basis of understanding."[19]

⌒

Rei-Ki-Balancing®

Another technique based upon the Usui System of Reiki is the *Rei-Ki-Balancing®* developed by Gerda E. Drescher. An essential component of the system that she developed in the late 1980s is the grounding work in which the energetic attunements on the feet play an important role. Gerda E. Drescher writes the following on this topic:

"I developed Rei-Ki-Balancing® through my many years of experiences as a therapist and healer, refining it and optimizing it in the course of a number of steps. As a body therapist and naturopath, I learned the Usui System of Natural Healing in 1983. I then had the first official Reiki practice in Germany until 1987. As a result of the comprehensive experiences gathered in countless Reiki treatments, I discovered that in many people the intensified flow of life energy resulting from the Reiki initiation is inadequately anchored on the physical level. With the grounding work according to the bioenergetic approaches and additional foot openings, I attempted to integrate the lower pole of the person into the Reiki energy work since in my experience this was not taken into consideration in the traditional Reiki teachings according to Hawayo Takata. At the same time, I discovered that the energy flow was even generally intensified through the foot openings."[20]

Polarities

An essential component in the philosophy of *Rei-Ki-Balancing®* is the thought that the *Ki,* as a part of the "Reiki", is an energy that ultimately always occurs in polar structure in its various forms:

"The term *Ki* (also called Chi or Qi) is used in different ways. Sometimes it is understood to be the entire life energy, and sometimes it primarily indicates that portion of it that flows through us as individuals and makes life possible for us on the earth in the material existence. The reason for the confusion about the term is that the universal life energy may be more or less individualized in its variety of forms, yet still remains an undivided whole on a deeper level. It is therefore helpful for our purposes to use the widespread Japanese expression of Reiki for the universal life energy and differentiate between the aspects of *Rei* and *Ki.* Here the *Rei* represents the omnipresent universal, unlimited potential, the original source, the undivided, non-manifested whole. *Ki* stands for the shaping aspect of the life energy, for example, that is individualized in a human being and together with the *Rei* affects the part of the whole represented by this person. While the Rei is unipolar and always remains unchanged, the *Ki* differentiates itself more and more in the countless forces and energy structures with polar character (yin—yang, upper pole—lower pole, Higher Self—Lower Self, light—shadow, good—evil, etc). (…) As the name of the method expresses, it is the goal of Rei-Ki-Balancing® to achieve a balance between the *Rei* and the *Ki.*"[21]

"Our experiences show," according to Gerda E. Drescher, "that in the traditional Reiki according to Hawayo Takata with the openings in the upper area, a strengthening or emphasis on the upper pole takes place. This can result in a shift in the equilibrium of the forces. It can lead the respective person feeling 'spacey' or 'floating.' The lower pole is pushed upward in the process, which worsens the grounding. The energy can then hardly be brought down to the ground anymore. This floating can lead to an ego inflation that frequently becomes noticeable in connection with the 3rd Degree initiation. The respective person then believes that he or she is very spiritual and advanced in development, not noticing how the suppressed shadow grows more and more with the increasing spiritual orientation. The earth connection of Rei-Ki-Balancing® strengthens the connection to the lower pole, improving the grounding as a result and therefore prevents the spaciness or floating. The tension is then increased at both poles, like a scale that stays balanced by adding weight to both sides of it."[22]

Module System

The system of *Rei-Ki-Balancing®,* according to Gerda E. Drescher, is built "upon the traditional Usui System of Natural Healing. Because of the additional energetic attunements (initiations are not done on the feet—they are exclusively associated with the upper pole), as well as through personal practitioner and teacher training, Rei-Ki-Balancing® is simultaneously a system of its own. However, the heart of the tradition according to Hawayo Takata, with the three levels of initiation and the corresponding integration periods, remains completely intact within the Rei-Ki-Balancing®. The content and structure of the training are not static but are adapted to the changing requirements of the collective process of transformation when necessary. This is simple in as far as it involves a closed module and a type of module system. At the same time, the previous knowledge of those who are interested plays a role in how their course of training is structured in terms of content and time. People who are already initiated into Reiki can receive the yin-yang balancing through the opening in the lower pole without having to attend an additional Reiki seminar."[23]

Life Path

Gerda E. Drescher received her Reiki training from Mary McFadyen and Phyllis Furumoto. At the beginning of 1986, she was initiated into the Master Degree by Phyllis Furumoto. In the following period of time, she taught the Usui System of Reiki in Italy, Germany, and Switzerland. Starting in 1994, she lived and worked in Switzerland where she founded the HoloEnergetic Lightbody Academy together with her husband, Edwin Zimmerli. In addition to the Usui System of Reiki and *Rei-Ki-Balancing®*, the couple also taught "various other methods for awakening the Lightbody (HoloEnergetic, Body-Clearing, Starcon, Metamorphing)"[24]. Within the "context of Lightbody awakening," they have also developed "an expanded understanding of Rei-Ki-Balancing®"[25].

On August 17, 2003 Gerda E. Drescher passed away after a brief disease at the age of 54 years. Her work is continued today by her husband, Edwin Zimmerli.

Regular Practice

As also in traditional Reiki as taught by Hawayo Takata, according to Gerda E. Drescher the daily practice for *Rei-Ki-Balancing®* is "treating yourself as often as possible, at best every day. All of the many spiritual possibilities do not replace the physical laying-on of hands."[26]

Furthermore, according to Edwin Zimmerli, there are special exercises that are a component of the practice such as the one on page 116 called "Bipolar Energy Flow." Part of the exercise is the energetic work with the eighth chakra, which is located about 18 to 22 centimeters (7 to 9 inches) above the center of the head.[27]

Bipolar Energy Flow
By Edwin Zimmerli

1. Stand comfortably. The feet should be about shoulder-width apart, and the spinal column is straight.

2. Open the knees somewhat so that the legs are no longer completely straight and the lower part of the pelvis tips forward very slightly. Make sure that your spinal column forms a vertical line. Let your breath flow freely and generously. If necessary, loosen your belt so the breath can also flow into the lower belly.

3. Sense your feet and the connection with the earth that carries you. Imagine that you are a tree of light. Powerful roots penetrate deep into the earth from your feet.

4. Now also feel your upper pole and imagine that branches, twigs, and leaves are growing out of your trunk far into the heavens and absorbing cosmic light.

5. Breathe conscious crystalline light from the earth into yourself through your roots and foot chakras. Allow it to travel up your legs to your heart. Let this light extend from there into all of your cells. Feel your grounding in the earth forces and your physical presence in the here and now. Take a few more breaths in this way and sense how the feeling of physical presence, power, and vitality is intensified.

6. Now breathe the cosmic light into yourself through your leaves, twigs, and branches from the eighth chakra above your head down to the crown chakra and further down into the heart center. Allow this cosmic light to spread from here into all of the cells. Feel your cosmic connection, your spiritual origin that inspires you and safely guides you through life. Take a few more breaths in this way and sense how a feeling of lightness and deep trust arises.

7. Be aware that you as a human being are the mediator and self-aware meeting point of heaven and earth. Spirit and matter, the rising and descending streams of consciousness meet within you. In your imagination, now let the crystalline light of the earth and the cosmic light of heaven simultaneously ascend and descend within you so that a continuous bipolar flow of energy is produced. As you do this, direct your attention to the central light channel that goes through your center

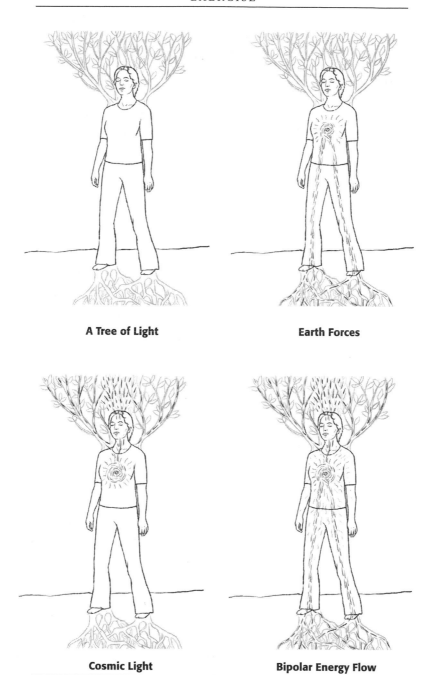

A Tree of Light

Earth Forces

Cosmic Light

Bipolar Energy Flow

and connects you with the higher, transpersonal chakra above your head. Sense how a feeling of pulsating light waves gradually arises.

8. Speak the following affirmation and feel its power: I am heaven and earth—I am unity—I am light!

Tip: This exercise can also be used for power-place work in order to specifically support the anchoring of the oneness/Christ consciousness on the earth.

New Approach to Reiki

Rei-Ki-Balancing®, according to Edwin Zimmerli, stands for "a new approach to the Reiki power" that supports "the bipolar flow of prana in the lightbody field is taken into consideration" and "the process of becoming whole through integrating the shadow".[28] So *Rei-Ki-Balancing®* helps the individual with the process of integrating the shadow, which was emphasized by C. G. Jung. By means of an expanded, bipolar approach, it follows the same goal as the Integral Yoga of Sri Aurobindo.[29]

"The bipolar energy attunements of Rei-Ki Balancing®," according to Edwin Zimmerli, "affect a developmental process in which the individual increasingly comes into contact with his true, multi-dimensional self. He/She becomes livelier, more flexible, and energetically more transparent. This promotes the abilities to express oneself and create boundaries. The old, assumed judgments and valuations, distorted self-images and projections are relativized by a higher perspective and ultimately fall away like the plaster of an old house. During the course of this process of purification and becoming conscious, the person begins to recognize his or her divine co-creative power, using it specifically for the benefit of all, and assume the full responsibility for his or her reality. He/She becomes free of guilt feelings and projections."[30]

Osho Neo-Reiki

Like *Rainbow Reiki* and *Rei-Ki-Balancing®*, *Osho Neo-Reiki* is another system based on the Usui System of Reiki according to Hawayo Takata that has been created by a German Reiki Master.

Osho Neo-Reiki was developed in the 1990s near the Indian Master Osho (formerly Bhagwan) by Himani H. Gerber. This occurred while she lived for a longer period of time in the "Mystery School" of the Osho commune in Puna (India), where she also taught Reiki.[31] Himani says that the day she gave her first Reiki seminar in the commune, she received a message from Osho:

"On the first day during my very first group, when I received the message from Osho: 'From now on call it Osho Neo-Reiki,' it was a great moment for me. How could I fulfill this name? What was my very personal song in this existence?"[32]

Many years before this time, Himani H. Gerber had already found her Master in Osho. Shortly thereafter, her history also began with Reiki: In 1982, she received her First Degree from Mary McFadyen and the Second Degree followed one year later. After a number of years of intensive experience with Reiki, she finally received the Master Degree in 1989, which was also from Mary McFadyen.[33]

The First Degree

At a seminar for the First Degree of *Osho Neo-Reiki,* according to Himani, four initiations are given.[34] The following contents are imparted:

"The weekend of a First Degree begins with an introduction to the topic of 'energy' and the history of Reiki, with information about the present currents. The approx. 20 basic positions for treating another person and the seven positions for self-treatment (corresponding with the seven energy centers in the body) are shown and practiced. In addition, a short treatment for harmonizing these energy centers (chakras) and their location in the body is taught. Furthermore, the first explanations about the various qualities of the chakras and their possible expressions in the personality are given.

Fundamental information on the topic of 'disease and healing' can help to bring more light and understanding into the emotions or thought patterns that are the basis of a symptom."[35]

Moreover, a seminar on the First Degree includes an introduction to two active meditation techniques according to Osho: the Osho Dynamic Meditation and the Osho Kundalini Meditation.[36] In her currently unpublished manuscript entitled "Neo-Reiki—New Dimensions of Your Transformation and Creativity," Himani explains:

"These meditations usually begin with intense activities such as hopping, breathing, or dancing. They are structured into various phases and have accompanying music that was created especially for these techniques under Osho's personal supervision. Only when the energies of the human body/mind system are activated, a silent phase follows in which the same energies can turn inward to the peaceful center, to the inner stillness."[37]

The Second Degree

According to Himani, three initiations are given at a seminar for the Second Degree of *Osho Neo-Reiki*[38]. The following contents are imparted:

"During a weekend with the Second Degree, there are detailed instructions on the practice of the Reiki symbols, as they were given by Mrs. Takata to Mary McFadyen. In my personal understanding, the first symbol effects a strengthening of the energy to be given; and it awakens my own potential of powerful (fire) energy. I introduce the Second Symbol specifically for spiritual healing (which means healing through the levels of consciousness). As the tradition has taught me, it creates within the recipient a bridge between the normal mind and the levels of sub- and supra consciousness; and within

121

myself, it causes a clear perception of this level of consciousness. The third symbol teaches us how we can give others Reiki distant treatment; and how we can develop more consciousness in the projection of energies in thought or emotions onto others."[39]

Furthermore, Himani writes about the techniques of the Second Degree:

"During the trainings for the Second Degree, we practice these new techniques and discuss and research the theoretical background of the seven levels of consciousness as the framework for spiritual healing, which means healing through the layers of the spirit/the mind. We frequently encounter hesitation about using these new techniques or even the fear of what is possible with them. Then it is time to give these inner processes their space and find the theme behind them; this often turns out to be the 'misuse of power in a past life.' When we come across the topic of misuse, it is good to remember that the knowledge of such a possibility already gives more attention to it—and so there is already a lower probability of engaging in further cases of misuse because of unconsciousness in the future. It is my feeling that the steps on the path inward is to discover the 'criminal corner' of the mind, where misuse, tyranny, and power struggles have already taken place."[40]

The techniques of the Second Degree, according to Himani, are "quite a large treasure chest with strong tools that are not all used at the same time but can be researched and integrated step by step. So many different layers want to be discovered. These will open up to the practitioners by themselves in harmony with the level of consciousness and the extent of the possible understanding."[41]

Training in Metaphysical Energy Work

As Himani writes, she has also developed the Trainings in Metaphysical Energy Work based on her experiences with the Reiki techniques, the inspiring insights of Osho, the observations in her personal process, and the perceptions of energetic changes on the part of many of her companions on the path. These are open to anyone who has a corresponding Reiki Degree.[42] The trainings are taught in three levels: Among other things, the first section offers structures that are intended to awaken and promote the perception and expansion of the spiritual heart space in the participants. In the second part, primarily the individual use of the symbol techniques of the Second Degree are compared with each other in an experimental manner with the goal of becoming more conscious in terms of the processes that take place within the practitioners on a subtle level. In part three, the abilities awakened in the second part are intensified, together with an exploration of inner attitudes and identifications such as the "helper," the "healer," and the "master."[43]

Master Degree

In terms of the initiation into the Master Degree of *Osho Neo-Reiki,* Himani writes:

"Those who received the Osho Neo-Reiki Master Degree from me usually already had contact with me through the years, contributed to the work in the commune or in some other work in the West or East. They had participated in the advanced training and used the time to practice on this level. They had also gone through their own and individual process and had used other methods and other groups and trainings for their personal transformation. Seen from my standpoint, the Master Degree is a certain completion of an inner process, which is also a process between the Reiki Teacher and the Reiki students. It is obviously also—and even more so—a new opening for a continuing process with Reiki, with the universal life force. A movement into new dimensions, from the work on oneself, to the work with others, to the work for the work. On the personal level, awakening is possible in order to become the master of oneself."[44]

Furthermore, she writes that the actual training for the Master Degree then lasts "three days, as energetic preparation, as a time for instruction and sharing, for meditating together, until the last initiation can take place as the climax of celebration and gratitude."[45]

Regular Practice

For the daily practice of *Osho Neo-Reiki,* Himani recommends a brief and very effective form of energy treatment that directly treats all of the seven chakras. This form of treatment bears the name of Osho Instant Reiki because it has an immediate effect on the energy system of human beings.[46]

For this book, Himani has selected the exercise on page 125, which she recommends for Reiki practitioners of all schools.

Reiki Jin Kei Do

According to Dr. Ranga Premaratna, *Reiki Jin Kei Do* is the name of a Reiki style whose spiritual lineage does not lead through Mrs. Takata. Instead, it goes from Dr. Hayashi to two Buddhist monks to him, the current lineage holder. Dr. Ranga Premaratna first used the name *Reiki Jin Kei Do* in 1997 with the goal of establishing a clear term for the system developed from this lineage.[47]

Feeling the Heart Space
By Himani H. Gerber

Hold your hands, with the palms in the direction of your body, in front of your chest at a bit of a distance. At a certain distance from your physical body, you can already feel an energetic connection here with your heart chakra, especially the outer layers.

Now let your hands slowly come closer to your chest and perceive the various energies as you do so. Also observe the different feeling that you may touch in the process. This may be a layer of pain—allow it—or a wave of sadness—feel it—or a feeling of expansiveness—observe it. In this way, you slowly come closer and closer until your hands actually touch your body.

With the Reiki touch, you will immediately perceive an energetic connection. Stay with it for a while until your energy hands are ready to stretch out. Allow them to melt into your physical body. Light hands can also reach inside. Your energy hands can melt into your chest toward the back. Without any effort, let it happen. Become conscious of the space within and its quality.

We always associate love with the heart, but we could also call it peace or trust, or? What is your word for this inner space?

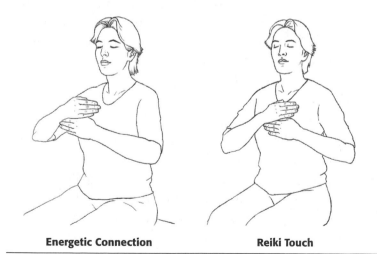

Energetic Connection   **Reiki Touch**

Gordon Bell, a teacher of *Reiki Jin Kei Do,* has explained the meaning of the Japanese words *Jin, Kei,* and *Do* as follows:

"Jin is the Japanese word for compassion and represents the Buddhist concept of universal compassion known as 'Karuna' in Sanskrit. Karuna is one of the fruits of deep spiritual training.

Kei is Japanese for wisdom, and represents Buddhist understanding of universal wisdom known as 'Prajna' in Sanskrit. Prajna is another fruit of deep spiritual practice.

Do is Japanese for 'way' or 'path' (Tao in Chinese), and links the ideas that Reiki is truly a path of spiritual development that integrates healing and meditation."[48]

In his article on "Reiki Jin Kei Do—The Path of Compassion and Wisdom through Reiki," Gordon Bell describes the path that this lineage took:

"Reiki Jin Kei Do is a lineage or style of traditional Reiki practice emphasizing the path of Reiki as a spiritual development with health supportive characteristics. It is sometimes known as 'Usui Shin Kai'—the 'core' or 'heart' teachings of Usui. (...) Its philosophy is grounded in the traditional views of Reiki, and like much of the Reiki taught and practiced in the West, it shares Mikao Usui and Chujiro Hayashi in its lineage. (...) Venerable Takeuchi received training from Dr. Chujiro Hayashi. (...) Dr. Hayashi did transmit form and teachings of Reiki to Venerable Takeuchi that included a series of meditations, said to be those Usui had practiced on Mount Kurama. (...) Venerable Takeuchi was an abbot of a small remote Zen temple where he administered Reiki to his followers. One student, Venerable Seiji Takamori, who entered the monastery at 19 years of age, later asked to be taught this practice. Over a period of 3 years, Venerable Takamori received training through the 3 levels or degrees of Reiki and he too helped in administering to the followers.

Venerable Seiji Takamori was instrumental in bringing this line of Reiki teachings to the West. Some time after he received training he asked his teacher Venerable Takeuchi, if he could leave the monastery and go on a search for further teachings relating to Reiki and Buddhist practices. With permission he embarked on a quest that would lead him through the Buddhist countries of Asia. In an isolated part of Nepal, he came across a small order of monks whose practice included a discipline similar to Reiki. This ancient system of healing contained two of the Reiki symbols and echoed the Buddhist teachings he was given by Sensei Takeuchi. Venerable Takamori decided to stay and study with three of the monks and was directed to a more advanced monk further into the Himalayas, whom he studied with for 7 years, receiving the deepest training on his progress to enlightenment. Contained within the training, were practices, teachings and symbology that paralleled the teachings he had received from Venerable Takeuchi, but that were more extensive. Thus he concluded, Usui had connected with the same stream of Buddhist teachings."[49]

Buddho Methods

The teachings that Seiji Takamori reportedly was given by the monks in the Himalayas are also called the Buddho Methods by practitioners and teachers of *Reiki Jin Kei Do*. Dr. Ranga Premaratna and other teachers of this tradition of Buddho Methods now also use the name EnerSense in addition to *Reiki Jin Kei Do*. As *Reiki Jin Kei Do* teacher Jim Frew explains in an article:

"Ranga now refers to the Buddho Method as the EnerSense System of Natural Healing. The word EnerSense is made from the words Energy, Sensation, and Sense."[50]

EnerSense, according to Gordon and Dorothy Bell, is a complete, health promoting system combining ancient Tibetan and Indian healing methods.[51] It includes meditative practices such as breath exercises that lead to meditative states of deep contemplation. *Chi-Nadi* exercises promote an advanced consciousness of energy, as well as self-healing by means of meditation and symbols, through the laying-on of hands, and with the breath.[52]

As Jim Frew has established, Dr. Ranga Premaratna believes that although there are direct links between Reiki and the Buddho System of Healing, it may not necessarily be the only origin of Reiki. The original sutra, which describes a healing method, could be interpreted differently by different monks depending on their own state of enlightenment. This could lead to the existence of more than one origin of Reiki.[53]

The Path to the West

Here is the continuation of the path of this Reiki lineage in the words of Gordon Bell:

"After completing his studies in the Himalayas, and with his teacher's blessing, Venerable Takamori continued his travels for study and teaching. His goal was to develop the healing system and his own mind, whilst helping others on his long journey. (...) During his travels Venerable Takamori had heard of another teacher (master) of Reiki in the West called Hawayo Takata, who had studied with his teacher's teacher, Dr. Hayashi, so in the early 1970's whilst in the West he met her."[54]

Dr. Ranga Premaratna explains: "Seiji Takamori was not a student of Hawayo Takata. He met her and received master initiation from her in exchange for his services as a monk. The reason Seiji requested the initiation from Takata was not because he needed training but to experience the energy transmission and information from another student of Hayashi, as his own teacher Ven. Takeuchi had received."[55]

"The Venerable Takamori", according to Gordon Bell, "continued travelling and teaching wherever he was requested and would be supported by those requesting teachings. Eventually in 1990 he transmitted his line of Reiki teaching and the additional studies (now including the quintessence of the Vajrayana Buddhist Yogic Tradition) to Dr. Ranga Premaratna PhD in the USA. Later, as Ranga Premaratna explored and practised the intensive training, he began teaching what was to become Reiki Jin Kei Do—the modern title for the lineage and teachings."[56]

As Jim Frew writes, before Dr. Ranga Premaratna met Seiji Takamori, he had already been initiated into all three degrees of Reiki.[57] Dr. Ranga Premaratna states that he received his earlier training in Reiki from Elke Petra Balm and Beth Sanders.[58] However, according to Jim Frew, Dr. Ranga Premaratna felt some of the information that he was given was incomplete once he had finished this training. As a result, he asked in the course of his meditation that one day he might meet the right teacher for him. He found him finally in Seiji Takamori.[59]

The Training

The general format of training in *Reiki Jin Kei Do,* according to Gordon Bell, follows the usual structure of traditional Reiki according to Usui: "Three degrees of training, four attunements at 1st Degree, one at 2nd Degree, and one at 3rd Degree. It is seen as a complete system, each level complete in itself, not requiring any prerequisite for commencement of training, but each level being the prerequisite for the next level of study. The lineage guidelines state that the training have a minimum of 3 months after 1st Degree and two years after 2nd Degree. Training at the first two degrees is over a minimum of two days, with additional course study, practice and feedback. At 3rd Degree the training is over 1 year. Practitioners of Reiki Jin Kei Do operating as Reiki Therapists are required to follow codes of Ethics, subject to local variations. E.g. here in the U.K. we have adopted the code of ethics of the UK Reiki Federation of which we are members."[60]

Within the scope of the First Degree, the students are introduced to "a form of practice of hand-on treatment for self and others; meditation practice and 'meditation with the hands' during Reiki practice; methods of self-awareness developing the ideals of Reiki; energy exercises to assist the student to fine-tune awareness of the flow of Reiki."[61]

"At Second Degree, the first three symbols of Reiki are presented with a deep level of insight and understanding of their background, meaning, and functionality. (…) Further treatment forms are used for self and others incorporating the body's energy fields, energy points (marma/tsubo) and energy pathways (nadi/meridian) and include absentia Reiki, continued development of meditation practice and self-reflexion."[62]

"At 3rd Degree, the fourth symbol is explored through meaning, philosophy and practice. Additional studies of energy systems, both theoretical and practical enhance the deeper experience of the flow of Reiki within. As progress is made, the syllabus of 1st and 2nd degree is studied in depth simultaneously with their respective attunements. After at least one year of practice and teaching, the Master attunement is studied and perfected and the year's practice is reviewed."[63]

One essential difference in the teachings of *Reiki Jin Kei Do,* according to Gordon Bell, is "the attention to the detail in the attunements. In *Reiki Jin Kei Do,* attunement is performed one-on-one. To prepare the body/mind for activation/tuning care is taken to balance the body energy and assess throughout the process of attunement the effectiveness of the attunement. Consequently, each attunement may last around 30 minutes per person. One of the repercussions is that training classes are often quite small, perhaps up to 4 trainees per initiating master."[64]

The exercise on page 132 is a fundamental component of the exercise cycle The Seven Purifying and Strengthening Breaths[65], which are an essential part of the practice of *Reiki Jin Kei Do.* This exercise is usually taught within the scope of a *Reiki Jin Kei Do* First Degree seminar and is presented in the instructions by Dr. Ranga Premaratna.

The Reiki Ideals

Within the teachings of *Reiki Jin Kei Do,* a special version of the Principles, called the Ideals of *Reiki Jin Kei Do,* are applied. This is "inspired by the copy of the ideals on Usui's memorial stone at Saihoji temple in Tokyo, and through the mind of wisdom and understanding of the practice of Reiki expressed by Venerable Seiji Takamori and Dr. Ranga Premaratna PhD."[66]

"Be mindful each moment of your day:

– To observe the arising of greed, anger and delusion, looking deeper for their true cause.
– To appreciate the gift of life and be compassionate to all beings.
– To find the right livelihood and be honest in your work.
– To see within the ever changing nature of your mind and body.
– To merge with the universal nature of the mind as Reiki flows within you."[67]

Harmonious Inner Communication

By Dr. Ranga Premaratna

1. Treating the crown (Washing the hair)

Stand with feet, one shoulder width apart, with knees slightly bent, the body relaxed, your hands down to the sides. Visualise that there is a pool of energy that looks like liquid silver in front of you. Raise your hands to the front of you, at the level of your navel, dip into this pool and take two handfuls of this liquid silver energy. Take a deep breath and imagine, as your hands are raised toward your head, that the liquid energy turns into two silver balls of energy pulsating with life. Bring your hands towards your forehead and move them slowly over your head, as if washing your hair. As your hands move down behind your head, stop for a few seconds at the base of the skull. Then, as you slowly exhale, bring your hands down to the starting position.

2. Treating the third-eye (Washing the face)

Start as in Point 1, but bring your hands toward your face as if washing the face. Leave palms about an inch from your face and focus on the sensations in the palms and the face. As you exhale, bring arms down to the starting position.

3. Treating the throat (Washing the throat)

Start as in Point 1, but bring your hands toward your throat as if washing the throat. Leave palms about an inch from your throat and focus on the sensations in the palms and the throat. As you exhale, bring arms down to the starting position.

4. Treating the heart (Washing the heart)

Start as in Point 1, but bring your hands to the chest, hold for a few seconds, separate palms by moving palms away from each other, and say to yourself: "Amplifying this energy of compassion within my heart." As your palms reach your shoulders, start exhaling and turning palms outward, as if pushing the balls of energy outward. Say to yourself: "Sharing this compassionate energy with all beings."

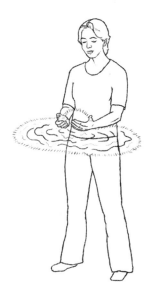

A Pool of Energy

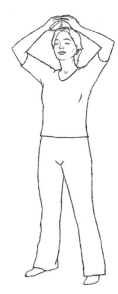

Energetic Cleansing

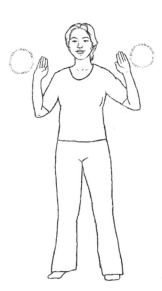

"Sharing this Compassionate Energy with All Beings"

Reiki Jin Kei Do and Buddho EnerSense

Anyone who would like to learn the Buddho-EnerSense Methods in addition to *Reiki Jin Kei Do,* can do this in the following way according to Gordon and Dorothy Bell:

"The normal route of study through the Lineage of Takamori and Buddho-EnerSense© is as follows: Reiki Jin Kei Do I, Reiki Jin Kei Do 2, EnerSense© I, EnerSense© II, Reiki Jin Kei Do 3, EnerSense© III, and EnerSense© IV. However, for those who have already taken Reiki 1, 2, and/or 3 in another lineage, we suggest the following: Reiki Jin Kei Do 1 and 2 attunements, EnerSense© I, Reiki Jin Kei Do 2 review, EnerSense© II, Reiki Jin Kei Do 3, EnerSense© III and EnerSense© IV. Buddho-EnerSense© is a continuation of studies in the Eastern Lineage of Takamori: Reiki Jin Kei Do©, therefore, re-attunement to Reiki Jin Kei Do 1 and 2 is necessary before commencing Buddho-EnerSense© training. Reiki Jin Kei Do 1 and 2 attunements can be given on an evening before the first training day."[68]

Jim Frew, who had already received the complete training in the Takata/Furumoto lineage (with his Master initiation in 1991) before his training in this system, describes his process with *Reiki Jin Kei Do* as follows:

"So why, people may ask, did I feel drawn to Ranga's lineage? Was I dissatisfied with my previous training? Definitely not! Did I believe I was learning something more 'powerful,' a 'better' form of Reiki? Definitely not! Was I satisfied with the authenticity of the information and the material that I had received? Yes; the integrity of the teachings was tangible and I intuitively knew that I followed an authentic path. Perhaps I was not able to authenticate the concrete facts of this lineage based on other sources, but I also did not try to do this since I was trained in the individual degrees of the Takata/Furumoto lineage. In these early years, I never had any reason to mistrust my teachers or my instincts. And there is much information that belongs to both of the lineages."[69]

⌒

Karuna Reiki®

Karuna Reiki® is a Reiki system developed by William Lee Rand on the basis of channeled symbols and is accessible only to Reiki Masters and teachers. After the initiation into the Master Degree and the corresponding teaching experience, it offers a possibility for deepening the path with Reiki. This occurs with the use of channeled materials and by working with spiritual guides.

William Lee Rand received the First and Second Reiki Degree in the early 1980s from Bethel Paigh. Some years later, he received trainings and initiations into the Master Degree from a total of four Reiki Masters: in 1989 from Diane McCumber and Marlene Schilke, in 1990 from Cherie Prasuhn, and in 1992 from Leah Smith. Shortly thereafter, he established the International Center for Reiki Training in Southfield, Michigan. William Lee Rand is the publisher of the American Reiki magazine *Reiki News* and author of several books on Reiki.[70] He write the following about the formative phase of *Karuna Reiki®* in an article:

"I became a Reiki Master in 1989 and soon began teaching full-time. After a few years, some students began showing me healing symbols that were not from the Usui System, nor were they from the Tibetan system of healing I had also learned. Because of this, I paid little attention to them. But after a while, other of students of mine began asking me about these non-Usui symbols and wanted to know what I knew about them. Eventually they began asking and eventually insisting that I create a class to teach how to use them. At first, I was reluctant to do so, as I was skeptical about anything that was not a part of an established system of healing. However, I eventually grew curious and began to suspect that perhaps there might be some value to some of them. In the winter of 1993 I organized a meeting of some of my most sensitive and devoted students to help in the process of understanding these new symbols. We said prayers and sent Reiki to our project, asking that we be guided to the symbols and attunement methods that would have the greatest value."[71]

As William Lee Rand explains, he did not "channel any of the symbols used in what eventually became Karuna Reiki®, but simply began to experiment along with my students with the symbols others had channeled and given to me. We did not know we were creating a new system of Reiki until months later when we experienced that the healing energies began to increase in frequency and strength. At first, I wondered if this was possible, but after other sensitive healers confirmed that the healing energies we were working with were significantly different than Usui Reiki, I slowly came to accept that a new system of Reiki was developing. I thanked the Creator and asked what to do next. I was directed to give it a name and the name that came was Karuna. I had not heard of this name before, but found it in a spiritual book and knew it was the right name."[72]

Signal Fire

Karuna, according to William Lee Rand, is "a Sanskrit word that is used in Buddhism, Hinduism, and Zen. It means compassionate action and this is not an ordinary kind of compassion, but one that comes from an unbounded sea of love. This is the kind of compassion that when combined with wisdom can lead to enlightenment. And once enlightened, all those who have followed this path are compelled by the great love that has grown in their hearts to turn their attention toward reducing suffering and helping others to also become enlightened. The beings who have followed this path and reside in this unbounded sea of love have unlimited power and at the same time unlimited kindness. They have mastered Karuna and because of this are its emissaries. They act like beacons sending unlimited healing potential into every part of the Universe."[73]

Furthermore, William Lee Rand writes: "Some have wondered why I have chosen to call this system Karuna Reiki® when in fact it is not part of the healing system Dr. Usui created. One must remember that Reiki is a Japanese word that was in use long before Dr. Usui began to use it. In fact, in Japan, the word Reiki is not commonly associated with the Usui System of Natural Healing, but is simply a generic word that refers to the occult, to healing or to things relating to spirit. In addition, since Karuna Reiki® evolved out of my experience with Usui Reiki and since it does make use of the Usui master symbol in the attunement process and other methods from Usui Reiki, it is appropriate that it also be considered a system of Reiki."[74]

"More Light than Form"

In the fundamental work on *Karuna Reiki®* authorized by William Lee Rand, *The Book On Karuna Reiki®*, author Laurelle Shanti Gaia writes her feelings in connection with the *Karuna Reiki®* energy:

"My first impression of Karuna Reiki® was that it is a very serious energy. Karuna Reiki goes very deep, gently but quickly. When using or receiving Karuna Reiki I find myself vibrating at a rapidly increasing rate, I feel like I am more light than I am form. The first few times I received a Karuna treatment I felt myself rise out of my body, and I was taken into each of the symbols used."[75]

137

An essential aspect of the system, according to Laurelle Shanti Gaia, consists of working together with spiritual guides. This makes *Karuna Reiki®* a "powerful tool for discerning Divine Guidance"[76]. The "spiritual guides who work with Karuna Reiki® are highly evolved"[77]; these include "the spiritual master Avalokiteshvara" and the archangels.[78]

She also writes: "One thing that is important for us to know is that (spiritual) guides can come to us in a limitless number of forms, or with no form at all. Sometimes guides appear as a human, animal, angel, or light being. At other times guides may be simply swirling masses of energy or color that we sense or see in our mind's eye. I have guides that communicate with me through sensations in my body. For example, when feeling a particular type of tingling around my shoulders and arms, I have come to know this as a signal that one of my guides is working with me to teach me new ways to direct energy. Other guides communicate through telepathic messages, sound, scent or by initiating a strong sense of inner knowing within me."[79]

In addition to working with spiritual guides, the work with gemstones is also a part of *Karuna Reiki®*. Gemstones, according to Laurelle Shanti Gaia, "help to intensify specific qualities of Karuna Reiki energy."[80] In addition, treatments with *Karuna Reiki®* also use the practice of chanting.[81] While giving Reiki, various vowels are sung that correspond with certain body zones in their healing effects.

Symbols and Levels

The training structure of *Karuna Reiki®* is described by William Lee Rand as follows: "The system of Karuna Reiki® has two practitioner levels and two master levels although the two master levels are usually taught together in one class. In addition, a common way to teach Karuna Reiki® for those wanting the whole system is to teach the complete system in one three-day class. Since only those with Reiki master training are permitted to take the training, this is possible as previous experience has given them experience in giving treatments and attunements which allow the additional information in Karuna Reiki® to be more easily understood."[82]

Furthermore, he writes: "In a Karuna Reiki® class, each symbol is explained including how to draw them and what they are for. An attunement is given and practice time of 2 hours or more is taken so that each student can experience the use of each of the symbols during a treatment. How to use the symbols for chanting and toning including demonstration and practice is also included. In the master training, the master attunement is given and there is demonstration and practice time of several hours or more to practice giving the attunements. These are the basic aspects of a class and there are also many other activities including meditations, lectures, discussion and sharing."[83]

"The two practitioner levels," according to William Lee Rand, "have four treatment symbols each for a total of eight. Each of the eight treatment symbols brings with it a different frequency and a different way of helping the healing process. As an example, there is a symbol to reduce pain and prepare for deep healing, one to heal deeply, one to fill the client with love and comfort, two for grounding and manifesting, one to attune to the higher mind, one to become centered in one's personal power, and one to bring peace."[84]

As William Lee Rand mentions, some of the symbols applied in *Karuna Reiki®* are also used in other healing systems. Here are his comments on this topic: "People wondered how two systems can be so different if they both use some of the same symbols. Actually, in any system of Reiki, the power or healing energy of a symbol does

Preparing for a Reiki Attunement
By William Lee Rand

The following steps are optional. Follow them if you feel guided to do so:

1. Refrain from eating meat, fowl, or fish for three days prior to the attunement. These foods often contain drugs in the form of penicillin and female hormones, and toxins in the form of pesticides and heavy metals, that make your system sluggish and throw it out of balance.

2. Consider a water or juice fast for one to three days, especially if you already are a vegetarian or have experience with fasting.

3. Minimize your use of coffee and caffeine drinks or stop completely. They create imbalances in the nervous and endocrine systems. Use no caffeine drinks on the day of the attunement.

4. Use no alcohol for at least three days prior to the attunement.

5. Minimize or stop using sweets. Eat no chocolate.

6. If you smoke, cut back and smoke as little as possible on the day of the attunement.

7. Meditate for half an hour each day for at least a week using a style you know or simply spend this time in silence.

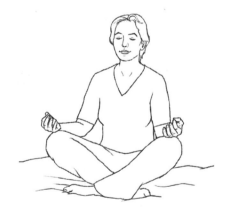

Meditation

8. Reduce or eliminate time watching TV, listening to the radio, and reading newspapers.

9. Go for quiet walks, spend time with nature, and get moderate exercise.

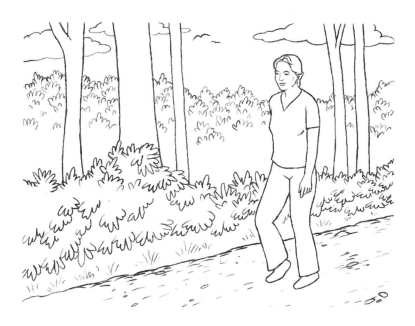

Walking in the Forest

10. Give more attention to the subtle impressions and sensations within and around you; contemplate their meaning.

11. Release all anger, fear, jealousy, hate, worry, etc., up to the light. Create a sacred space within and around you.

12. A Reiki attunement is an initiation into a sacred metaphysical order that has been present on Earth for thousands of years. By receiving an attunement you will become part of a group of people who are using Reiki to heal themselves and each other, and who are working together to heal the Earth. By becoming part of this group, you will also be receiving help from the Reiki guides and other spiritual beings who are working toward these goals.

not come from the symbol itself, but comes from the attunement or initiation. It is the attunement that actually empowers the symbol and attaches the healing energy to it. If one is using a different attunement method, then the energies being brought in and connected to the symbols will be different. A symbol in this case is very similar to a name. Two people can have the same name, but are still two distinctly different people."[85]

"There are no special hand positions with Karuna Reiki® that are different than in Usui Reiki. One can give a complete treatment using all the basic hand positions, or one can use one's intuition or a scanning method to be guided to the places where the client needs Reiki the most. Karuna Reiki® can also be used with Usui symbols. As an example, the Usui power symbol can be used with any of the Karuna Reiki® symbols. If one wants to send Karuna Reiki® at a distance, one can use the Usui distant symbol along with any of the Karuna Reiki® symbols to send it at a distance."[86]

Spiritual Way of Life

Since the practice of *Karuna Reiki®* is exclusively reserved for Reiki Masters and this book will also be read by practitioners of the First and Second Degrees, as well as people who are not even initiated into the Usui System of Reiki, it is not possible to include an exercise of the *Karuna Reiki®* system here. Furthermore, all of the exercises that are part of *Karuna Reiki®* contain mantras and symbols that are to be kept secret and cannot be published here (just as the symbols and terms of the Second Degree of the Usui System are not published in this book).

William Lee Rand has agreed to have an excerpt of his book *Reiki: The Healing Touch*[87] reproduced here. It comprehensively brings to mind all the points that are worth considering within the scope of a spiritual way of life. This list was created by William Lee

Rand as a collection of reference points for "Preparing for a Reiki Attunement." The fundamental idea is that, especially in the phase before a Reiki initiation, it can be advantageous to keep the body and mind pure in order to prepare it for the energetic processes that occur within the scope of initiation. In addition, this list can also be seen as a general collection of spiritually oriented behaviors. For those who orient themselves upon it within the scope of preparation for a Reiki initiation, it is especially important to only follow the advice that feels right and appropriate for them. The list on page 140 should also not be understood as a "must."

Other Styles

In addition to the five forms of the work with Reiki described here as examples that are based upon the Usui System, there are now many other Reiki styles. However, the majority of these, as far as I know, have not yet reached a larger area of influence. In *The Reiki Sourcebook* by Bronwen and Frans Stiene, for example, there is a list of about 40 different styles, whereby the authors have determined that even this list is probably still incomplete.[88] Among those styles that have not been mentioned in any other place in this book are: Alchemia Reiki, Angelic RayKey, Blue Star Reiki, Braha Satya Reiki, Dorje Reiki, Imara Reiki, Johrei Reiki, Lightarian Reiki, Mahatma Reiki, New Life Reiki, Reido Reiki, Reiki Plus, Reiki Tummo, Saku Reiki, Satya Reiki, Tara Reiki, Tera Mai Reiki, and Vajra Reiki.

However, it is difficult to determine whether this is a style with a specific area of validity that should be taken seriously or in some cases just the "proclamation" of a "new" important Reiki style on the part of a Reiki Teacher attempting to draw attention to his or her work without achieving resonance with a larger number of people. It would obviously be a foolish enterprise to become involved in the energy space of each individual, smaller Reiki style just for the purpose of research. However, I would like to say that some of the websites giving information about the founders of the above-mentioned styles and their respective approaches to Reiki—such as that of Kathleen Milner, the founder of *Tera Mai Reiki*—do trigger a certain sense of irritation within me in terms of the quality of the content and the argumentation.[89]

Consequently, I will abstain from providing information in this book about other styles of Reiki unknown to me. But this does not mean that I am judging the above-mentioned styles or the small Reiki styles that are not included in any way. Those who want more information about the smaller Reiki styles not discussed here can consult *The Reiki Sourcebook* by Bronwen and Frans Stiene.

The five forms of working with Reiki on the basis of the Usui System described extensively in this chapter are intended to be a representative, exemplary selection. In addition to the information about the forms described, these descriptions should also provide a fundamental understanding of the topic of further developments of spiritually oriented systems. In making my selection, I have taken into consideration the founders or lineage holders to whom I have personal contact and with whom I can feel a certain integrity in terms of their practice and teachings. Other forms of the work with the universal life energy based upon the Usui System of Reiki that claim a certain amount of validity here will be presented in Chapters 6 and 8.

Old and New

Each new form of the work with Reiki based on the Usui System has its origin in the unique path of one individual—just as the Usui System itself had its origin in the individual path of one person, namely in that of Mikao Usui. To which extent the experience of an individual on his or her own path is brought into a certain form that has significance that extends to other people and receives a larger degree of validity as a result can only be proved in the course of time.

Not every further development of an originally learned form must necessarily lead to the establishment of a new form. A further development is also possible within a form that already exists; however, this is certain to be in a much lesser degree and a much slower tempo than permitted by the establishment of a new form.

The establishment of a new form is sometimes preceded by a break with the (earlier) teacher and his or her teaching, above all when this person teaches a traditional form he or she does not believe should be changed. Such a break can be related to the (previous) student and now new founder being dissatisfied with which he or she has received, or at least finding it to be insufficient. As long as this does not lead to completely turning away from the practice but continuing to experience it as valuable, this type of situation is frequently the starting point for not only wanting to expand the received practice and teachings for oneself but also desiring to aim for a new, generally accessible form for "like-minded people". If conflicts should arise in this situation between the (earlier) teacher of the founder and the (previous) student of this teacher, who is now the founder of the new form, they should not forget that both participants are ultimately just playing their role in "the game of life." I believe that the key to resolving this kind of discord is simply in forgiveness on the part of both participants and in both directions.

The text on page 147 was written by Phyllis Lei Furumoto after I asked her for a contribution to this book. During my visit to Idaho in June 2004, I had explained the dimensions and aspects of this book. As a result, I received her support on various levels. I would like to thank her for this support and for her clear words in her text on "The Way with Reiki."

The Way with Reiki
By Phyllis Lei Furumoto

Since Hawayo Takata was able to practice Usui Shiki Ryoho in Hawaii and therefore, the United States, students have been exploring the effects of this practice in their lives. From the time of her death in 1 980, students have also been altering the form of the practice that she taught. Sometimes the changes came to fit the needs of the students, sometimes to fit the needs of the master, sometimes to reflect the life philosophy of the master, and sometimes through misunderstanding. This process is a natural one. When we, as humans, find something that opens the door to the self, the first thing we wish to do is make it our own. We do this by introducing our personal desire and philosophy into the practice.

As the process continues, the alterations and changes of the practice result in different forms of practice with different fundamental principles that guide the student in the practice. As a result, today there are many different forms of practice to choose from and to explore. These give students a variety of forms from which to choose. Eventually, a student will come to the place within that asks for a choice. What form serves me? Then the next step for a student is practice. Practice in two ways. Practice, as in practicing over and over again. Treating as much as possible, receiving treatments, applying the principles in daily life, and using the guidance of Reiki, the energy, in our lives. As the practice deepens I have found that it is the consistency of practice that creates the value and depth of a student's path.

At this point the student has chosen a form of practice, has spent time with the practice, and has surrendered to the process of living with the energy of Reiki. The application of the practice then permeates all aspects of life. This is the ultimate challenge for any spiritual practice; for any healing art. The deeper questions come to the surface.

How can I hold my practice as precious to me while letting others find a different practice? How can I respect and honor other masters when I don't agree with them? How can I find my own place in the world of spiritual commerce without denigrating others? Can I allow others to support me if I don't agree with them? How do I carry my path without comparing my path to someone else's?

What I have learned throughout my practice is that Reiki energy brings me into alignment with my natural path as a human being and as an individual. The more I am able to surrender to this path and no other, the more I am able to have peace and clarity that this is my path and no one else's. If others wish to learn the form I practice, I am willing to teach. This will give the new students a beginning point at which to develop their own path through the form of practice we share.

As a master I carry two principles within me. I have a right to my path and my private practice is not bound by form but by my development as a student. The second is as a master who teaches others, I have a responsibility to represent the form of the practice I hold and to present it to new students as simply and clearly as is possible. I am bound by my surrender to a practice that has held me and given me all that I need for my personal development.

Each of us who are living in this modern world with instant communication and choices of all kinds are faced with the dilemma of discernment. In the relative world, comparison assists us in making decisions. In the absolute world of spirit, there is no comparison possible. There is only choice. No choice is more right or wrong than another. So our task in these days is to let go of our need for relative world decisions and to embrace the sometimes confusing world of choice. Once we have made a choice, we can make another one. We can choose our master and our form at one time in our life. Should we need to make another choice, this also can be done. And with the choice there need not be blame, comparison of what is more traditional or authentic, nor the search for personal safety within the practice.

The wonderful thing is that we have the possibility of treating ourselves with Reiki when it is too confusing, when it becomes painful, when the healing is deep and fierce, when the joy overflows and the tears run down without cause. The miracle of being able to use this deep and inherent part of ourselves for the benefit of ourselves and others brings out the gratitude for a man, Mikao Usui and his quest. I trust that we all join in expressing our gratitude and awe for the gift that we hold in our hands naturally.

6. The Rediscovery
Back to the Roots!?

The discovery of the memorial stone for Mikao Usui at the Saihoji Temple in Tokyo in 1994 was a milestone in the recent history of the Usui System. After Frank Arjava Petter reported on it in his first book, *Reiki Fire,* which was first published by *Windpferd* in Germany and then went around the whole globe, the "Reiki world" was never the same. It initiated a process that is continuing in the course of which millions of Reiki Teachers and practitioners throughout the world reflected on their teachings and practice in the light of the newly gained perceptions, becoming increasingly conscious of the historical correlations. Many people have experienced the confrontation with this new information about Mikao Usui in a way similar to what Walter Lübeck writes in his preface to *Reiki Fire:*

"I am fascinated here by the figure of Dr. Usui, who has emerged in a totally unusual way for the most part. On the one hand, he is clearly no longer the magical, practically superhuman figure who appears to be perfect, but in another sense he gains immensely in human stature, and I find him much more likeable than back when it was only possible to learn something about him through strongly stylized stories that were passed on by word of mouth."[1]

Frank Arjava Petter

Frank Arjava Petter had written his book *Reiki Fire* in 1995 with the initial intention of publishing it in Japan, where he lived at that time with his wife Chetna Kobayashi.[2] At the end of 1992, when he was already living in Japan, he returned to Germany for a brief time in order to learn Reiki for himself. In the process, he received the initiations into all three degrees of the Usui System (from his brother), and at the beginning of 1993, he initiated his wife Chetna into Reiki when he returned to Japan. Although he originally had not planned to teach Reiki in Japan, Frank Arjava and Chetna already decided a few months later to offer all three Reiki degrees in Sapporo. Up to that time, as Frank Arjava Petter writes, it was only possible to learn the first two Reiki degrees in Japan. Consequently, many people who already had the First or Second Reiki Degree came to Sapporo to continue their Reiki training with Frank Arjava and Chetna.[3]

At about the same time, Frank Arjava and Chetna began their research on the origin of the Usui System. They located a direct relative of Mikao Usui, the wife of his grandson, but she did not want to say much about her husband's grandfather. As Frank Arjava writes, it sounded to him at that time as if Mikao Usui had had a falling out with his family or at least with some of the family members.[4] A short time later, one of Frank Arjava and Chetna's Reiki students who lived in Tokyo found the memorial stone and the grave of Mikao Usui at the Saihoji Temple at their request. Furthermore, this resulted in contacts to people who had information about the origin of the Usui System, including Mrs. Kimiko Koyama, who was president of the *Usui Reiki Ryoho Gakkai*[5] at that time, Mr. Fumio Ogawa, and Mr. Tsutomu Oishi:

"In August of 1995, our friend Shizuko Akimoto, who had learned Reiki from Chetna and with whom we work closely, met with Mr. Tsutomo Oishi, who had learned Reiki more than 30 years ago. Mr. Oishi had come to Shizuko, a wonderful healer, for a healing session. He suddenly began to speak about Reiki, without knowing that Shizuko is a Reiki teacher herself. Mr. Oishi introduced Shizuko to a Mr. Fumio Ogawa, whose adoptive father Kozo Ogawa had been a close colleague of Dr. Usui's and the chairman of the Reiki community in Shizuoka. As a result, more and more information came to light every week."[6]

As Fumio Ogawa reported, "for a while, Mikao Usui had been the private secretary of the politician Shimpei Goto, who was the Secretary of the Railroad, the Postmaster General, and the Secretary of the Interior and State. In the year Taisho 9 (1922), Mr. Goto became the mayor of Tokyo. We can also assume that Dr. Usui had good relations with many influential politicians and perhaps his travels outside of Japan, which he presumably embarked on according to the inscription on his tombstone, can be explained this way. However, we still do not know exactly what his duties were in the service of Mr. Goto."[7]

Furthermore, Tsutomo Oishi provided the following information: "During Dr. Usui's lifetime the local Reiki center in Shizuoka, was headed by a Mr. Kozo Ogawa. (...) Dr. Usui recognized Mr. Ogawa's healing talents and ultimately elevated him to the highest rank in the organization. Dr. Usui and Mr. Ogawa used to give energy-charged crystal balls to their students. These crystal balls were placed directly on the patient's diseased area, helping the body to find its equilibrium again. After initiation, all students also received a manual that explained what Reiki is, described symptoms and gave guidelines for the treatment of illnesses. People attending a Reiki meeting would kneel in the traditional Japanese style, fold their hands in front of their chest in the 'gassho' or 'namaste' position. The Reiki teacher would then touch the student's clasped hands with one hand and estimate their healing talent and energy."[8]

It has also been reported that Dr. Usui spoke respectfully about the Meiji Emperor.

Gassho Meditation
According to Mikao Usui, as instructed by Frank Arjava Petter

Gassho literally means "two hands coming together" and Dr. Usui taught a meditation by the name of Gassho Meditation. This meditation was practiced each time at the beginning of his Reiki workshops/meetings. It is meant to be practiced for 20-30 minutes after getting up and/or in the evening before going to sleep. Gassho can be done alone or in a group. Group meditations are a wonderful experience since the energy increases far beyond the sum of the individual participant's energies.

The Gassho Meditation is so simple that individuals of any age can do it. Whether we like it or not is another question. For my part, I love it very much and can also warmly recommend it. After three days of practice, you will know on the basis of your feelings whether it is "right" for you. Then, if possible, you should practice it every day for at least three months.

However, if after one or two days you have a feeling of restlessness, irritability, or some other form of annoyance, this meditation may possibly not be suitable for you. Not every medicine works for each patient. Then you can simply try it again after a few weeks.

Many people who are experienced in meditation know how difficult it is to forget everything and let go of our rational mind and the inner dialog. However, we tend to forget especially when we want to remember something! My tip is to disidentify yourself from your thoughts and feelings during meditation, as well as from your senses, but don't close yourself off to them. Whenever we try to close ourselves, this is when the inner dialog really starts up.

When doing Gassho, sit down with closed eyes and hands placed together in front of your chest. Focus your entire attention at the point where the two middle fingers meet. Try to forget everything else. If you begin to think about lunch or the coming day during this meditation, observe the thought and then let it go.

This is not a matter of achieving something. Relax as well as you can relax. Then return to the point where your middle fingers meet.

If it is painful for you to hold your hands folded together in front of your chest for 20 minutes, let your hands (keeping them together) slowly sink down to your lap into a comfortable position and continue to meditate.

Energy phenomena may also occur, such as your hands or backbone becoming very warm: Observe this but don't let yourself be influenced by it. Always return your focus to your two middle fingers.

If you must change your sitting position, then move in slow motion: deliberately and consciously. In my experience, it is easier to meditate when the spinal column is as straight as possible, and the head doesn't tilt either forward, backword, or to the side. Imagine that your head is attached to a balloon filled with helium, which gently keeps it in the perfect position. If you have back problems or aren't used to sitting, I recommend that you sit on a chair with a back, with a few pillows behind you, or with your back leaned against the wall. There are basically no objections to meditating while lying down except that it invites us to fall asleep.

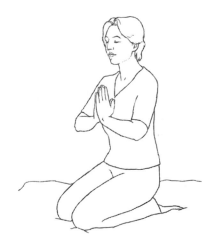

Gassho in Japanese Posture

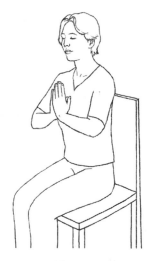

Gassho on a Chair

Gassho Meditation

In *The Original Reiki Handbook of Dr. Mikao Usui,* which was first published in Germany in 1999 by *Windpferd,* Frank Arjava Petter included the *Gassho* Meditation[9], which he called one of the "three pillars" of the Reiki System according to Mikao Usui. This is reproduced on page 152.

In *The Reiki Sourcebook,* Bronwen and Frans Stiene write the following about the *Gassho* Meditation:
"The *gassho* brings all opposites together. It creates unity within the body by bringing the left- and right-hand side together. All opposites become one. It is possible to see how focused an individual is by their *gassho.* If their concentration is poor, their *gassho* will be loose and sloppy. A firm *gassho* indicates a quiet and focused mind."[10]

Reiki Ryoho Hikkei

As Frank Arjava Petter writes in the preface to *The Original Reiki Handbook of Dr. Mikao Usui,* he and his wife Chetna received a copy of the *Reiki Ryoho Hikkei,* the "Handbook of the Reiki Healing Method" that dates back to Mikao Usui from Tsutomu Oishi in the summer of 1997.[11] He also writes that Tsutomu Oishi's mother learned the Reiki method of healing directly from Mikao Usui.[12] It appears that this handbook was given to every participant of a First Degree *(Shoden)* seminar.[13]

Doctrine

The "Handbook of the Reiki Healing Method" begins with a formal explanation by Mikao Usui of the *Usui Reiki Ryoho Kyogi.*[14] *Kyogi* means something like doctrine, which is a programmatic definition. Therefore, *Usui Reiki Ryoho Kyogi* means something like "the Doctrine of the Reiki Healing Method According to Usui." In this doctrine, Usui primarily explains why he publicly teaches the Reiki method of healing (cf. pg. 39).[15] Furthermore, the beginning of the handbook includes the five Principles in addition to the doctrine.[16]

Questions and Answers

The second part of the "Handbook of the Reiki Healing Method" consists of questions to Mikao Usui regarding the *Reiki Ryoho* and his answers to them.[17] As Bronwen and Frans Stiene have determined, the origin of this part of the handbook was probably the notes of some of Usui's students who had questions and wrote them down in their papers, as well as Usui's responses to them.[18] For example, Mikao Usui supposedly responded to the question "What is the *Usui Reiki Ryoho?*" in the following way:

"With thankfulness we receive and live according to principles (...) prescribed by the Meiji Emperor. In order to achieve the proper (spiritual) path for humanity, we must live according to these principles. This means that we must learn to improve our spirit and body with practice. To do this, we first heal the spirit. Afterwards, we make the body healthy. When our mind finds itself on the healthy path of honesty and seriousness, the body will become healthy completely on its own. So the mind and body are one, and we live out our life in peace and joy. We heal ourselves and the illnesses of others, intensifying and increasing our own happiness in life, as well as that of others. This is the goal of the *Usui Reiki Ryoho.*"[19]

In another of Usui's responses, it becomes clear that the practice of the *Reiki Ryoho* did not just consist of laying on of hands. For example, he asserts that the Second Degree, *Okuden*, consists of "a number of (healing) methods: *Hatsuleiho,* (light) tapping, stroking,

155

pressing with the hands, distance healing, the healing of the habits (mental healing), and so forth. (…)."[20] In another paragraph, Usui explains that the Reiki method of healing "uses neither medications nor instruments. It uses only looking, blowing, stroking, (light) tapping, and touching (of the afflicted parts of the body)."[21]

Frank Arjava Petter writes the following about this: "Without these techniques, it would not be possible to understand the intuitive bodywork of Dr. Usui: 1. He touched the diseased parts of the body. 2. He massaged them. 3. He tapped them. 4. He stroked them. 5. He blew on them. 6. He fixed his gaze on them for two to three minutes. 7. He specifically gave them energy. One Japanese Reiki school teaches that Dr. Usui received the Reiki energy with his left hand and passed it on with his right hand. He is said to have brought the fingertips of his left hand together with the thumb, as if he were holding a raw egg. The fingertips of the middle finger and ring finger of the right hand are said to have touched the tip of the right thumb. The little finger and the index finger were said to have stood away from the middle and ring finger at a ninety-degree angle."[22]

Treatment Plan

The third portion of the "Handbook of the Reiki Healing Method" consists of an overview of the standard hand positions for treating specific body parts and illnesses. This portion is called *Ryoho Shishin,* which means something like "Treatment Plan of the Healing Method" in English. Other possible translations are "Indications for Treatment with the Healing Method" or "Healing Method's Guideline."[23]

The *Ryoho Shishin* is subdivided into eleven chapters[24]:

1. Basic Treatment for Specific Parts of the Body
2. Functional Disorders of the Nerves

3. Functional Disorders of the Respiratory Organs (and Air Passages)
4. Functional Disorders of the Digestive Organs
5. Functional Disorders of the Circulatory (Cardiovascular) System
6. Functional Disorders of the Metabolism and the Blood
7. Functional Disorders of the Urogenital Tract
8. Operation Wounds and Functional Disorders of the Skin
9. Childhood Diseases
10. Women's Health
11. Contagious Diseases

As Bronwen and Frans Stiene write, there was probably a number of versions of set hand positions for the treatment of others that Mikao Usui taught at various times. These also include a sequence of five head positions that may constitute a type of basic treatment.[25] These five head positions are similar to some of the head positions found in *Ryoho Shishin,* Chapter 1, under the heading of "Basic Treatment for Specific Parts of the Body." However, a closer look reveals that the *Ryoho Shishin* does not contain any standardized form of the basic treatment for the treatment of others or for self-treatment.

As Frank Arjava Petter writes, Mikao Usui probably taught what was basically a type of "intuitive Reiki" that is primarily concerned with finding the *Byosen* (cf. pg. 45).[26] In a similar vein, Hiroko Kasahara states: "The *Byosen* can be found where the cause or source of the disease sits, and not always where the pain or the symptom manifests. The head is usually also included in the treatment since this is where the center of the powers of self-healing is located. However, a specific partial treatment is then usually done instead of a full-body treatment. Someone who cannot find the *Byosen* should lay his hand according to the *Reiki Ryoho Shishin* ("Guideline for Reiki Treatments"). This describes which body parts should be treated for which disease."[27]

Furthermore, Hiroko Kasahara states that Mikao Usui "with the exception of paired organs like the ears, lungs, and kidneys, usually gave treatments with just his right hand, in such a way that the middle section of his middle finger gently touched the area to be treated. At the same time, it is said that he probably frequently formed a circle with the index finger and thumb of his left hand; from here, he charged the energy."[28]

On the basis of their research, Bronwen and Frans Stiene conclude: "Self-treatment by placing hands on one's own body was not taught directly by Mikao Usui. The recitation of *Waka* and the five precepts along with the mantras and meditation techniques were the earliest forms of self-development taught to students."[29]

Yet, a closer look reveals that Mikao Usui apparently found self-treatment with Reiki to be important. In the second part of the "Handbook of the Reiki Healing Method," under the "Questions and Answers," it says:

"Question: With it (the *Usui Reiki Ryoho)*, other people can be healed. But what about oneself? Can a person also heal his own health disorders?

Answer: If we cannot heal our own diseases, then how should we heal others?"[30]

As I learned from Hiroko Kasahara, she heard that the current daily form of Reiki practiced by members of the *Usui Reiki Ryoho Gakkai* also includes an element of self-treatment in which a person treats himself in an intuitive manner, as described above, in addition to reciting the Reiki Principles and practicing the *Gassho* Meditation.[31]

Poems by the Meiji Emperor

The fourth and last part of the "Handbook of the Reiki Healing Method" consists of 125 poems by the Meiji Emperor, selected by Mikao Usui for the spiritual work (cf. pgs. 31–32). The poems by the Meiji Emperor in the *Waka* style, of which there supposedly were a total of 100,000, are called *Gyosei* in Japanese.[32] *Waka* is the name used for a traditional form of Japanese poetry and means "Japanese song." It consists of 31 syllables that are divided into five lines in the following way: 5-7-5-7-7. Hiroko Kasahara writes: "The first three lines (5-7-5) belong to the upper verse, which often serves as an introduction. The two last lines (7-7) belong to the lower verse, which serves as the conclusion. In the austere clarity of a brief, strict form, images, feelings, and moods are concentrated and expressed like a snapshot. The strong stylization of the moment condenses an abundance of intimations and fleeting references so that a *Waka* can contain a complexity or ambiguity."[33]

The 125 poems of the Meiji Emperor that Mikao Usui selected for the spiritual work are printed with an English translation in the book *The Spirit of Reiki* by Walter Lübeck, Frank Arjava Petter, and William Lee Rand. Here is one of the poems:

> Evening
>
> When the sun
> Begins to set
> I miss the day
> That I spent
> Idle[34]

(Additional poetry of the Meiji Emperor can be found in this book on pages 31 and 32.)

Dr. Hayashi's Treatment Plan

In addition to his books on the life and work of Mikao Usui, Frank Arjava Petter has also worked with Tadao Yamaguchi to create a book on Dr. Hayashi *(The Hayashi Reiki Manual)*. The contents of this book have already been described in chapter 2 (see pg. 38 f). A portion of this book is an additional version of the *Ryoho Shishin*, which dates back to Dr. Hayashi, this is the "Treatment Plan for the Healing Method" according to Dr. Hayashi.

As Frank Arjava Petter writes, the treatment plan by Dr. Hayashi is somewhat different than the one by Mikao Usui. For example, because Dr. Hayashi was a physician it contains many medical words.[35] However, since the difference between the two treatment plans are not that significant in terms of the hand positions, as Bronwen and Frans Stiene point out[36], we can assume that Dr. Hayashi was already involved in creating the first treatment plan together with his teacher Mikao Usui.[37]

The *Ryoho Shishin* according to Dr. Hayashi is divided into nine sections[38]:

Part 1: Head in general
Part 2: Diseases of Digestive Organs
Part 3: Respiratory Diseases
Part 4: Cardiovascular Diseases
Part 5: Urinary Organ Diseases
Part 6: Neurological Diseases
Part 7: Infectious Diseases
Part 8: Diseases of the Whole Body
Part 9: Other Diseases and Symptoms

Meditation Techniques

Before the Usui System of Reiki was passed on to Mrs. Takata by Dr. Hayashi, it apparently went through some changes in the hands of Dr. Hayashi. These changes probably included omitting most of the meditation techniques, which had been more at the center of the practice of the system during Mikao Usui's lifetime. This conclusion is supported by *The Original Reiki Handbook of Dr. Mikao Usui* (edited by Frank Arjava Petter) and *The Reiki Sourcebook* (Bronwen and Frans Stiene). Dr. Hayashi, according to the research by Bronwen and Frans Stiene, only passed on four or five of the original techniques to his students Hawayo Takata and Chiyoko Yamaguchi.[39] "This may mean that Chujiro Hayashi did not know them to pass on, did not place an emphasis on them, or the other techniques (those that Hayashi did not teach, author's note) were not introduced till a later date."[40]

Initiation Rituals

When I learned the initiation rituals for the First and Second Degree within the scope of my Master training in November 2000 from my teacher, Paul Mitchell, I sometimes asked myself the question: Are these actually the original forms of the initiation rituals as they were already done before us by Mikao Usui, Dr. Hayashi, and Mrs. Takata? Or did the form of the ritual change within the course of the decades? The background for this question was in no way doubt about the effectiveness of the rituals. To the contrary: I was certain and could also feel that the essence of these rituals has been preserved to the present as they were passed originally from Mikao Usui to Dr. Hayashi, from Dr. Hayashi to Mrs. Takata and from her to Paul Mitchell, my teacher. And, of course, they came to me in the form and through the teacher that was appropriate for me. Perhaps it was simply curiosity: the urge to reflect on things and become aware of the larger correlations.

Some years later, while researching this book, I came across some reflections by Bronwen and Frans Stiene in *The Reiki Sourcebook* indicating that Dr. Hayashi apparently made changes to the initiation ritual: "The attunement process that is performed today, in all its variations, utilizes mantras and symbols. This is not the case in the *Usui Reiki Ryoho Gakkai* or other traditional Japanese teachings where these methods of attunement are called *reiju* and are practiced without mantras and symbols. This is a major difference between what Chujiro Hayashi taught and Mikao Usui's teachings."[41]

Unfortunately, the references that are so numerous in the rest of this book are lacking at this point in *The Reiki Sourcebook*. Yet, these reflections are probably correct because there are also similar thoughts in the text of other authors such as Hiroko Kasahara. In her article on Reiki in Japan, she writes that on the basis of her knowledge about the current initiation practice of the teachers in the *Usui Reiki Ryoho Gakkai,* she assumes that Dr. Hayashi made changes in the initiation rituals.[42]

As we know today, Dr. Hayashi had a decisive influence on the Usui System before passing it on to Mrs. Takata. Consequently, it is not surprising that the initiation rituals also underwent some changes. If this is the case, it probably occurred with the goal of making the overall system more effective, which would once again underline Hayashi's special role that he played in shaping the Usui System in a way that really made it possible for it to spread throughout the world.

In an article in the *Reiki News Magazine,* Frank Arjava Petter writes about the role that Dr. Hayashi and Mrs. Takata played in the development of the Usui System of Reiki: "Reiki evolved differently in schools both inside and outside of Japan. By the time Hawayo Takata brought Reiki to the Western world, it had changed its face considerably. According to Hiroshi Doi (…), Dr. Hayashi with whom Takata had studied, was asked by Usui to develop a new style of *Reiki Ryoho* based on Dr. Hayashi's medical background. Hayashi did this and eventually left the *Gakkai*. This new style included changes in the hand positions, two or more giving Reiki treatments to one client, a different method of attunements, and teaching *Okuden* (Reiki II) in one 5 day class. This system was modified again by Takata in order to make it acceptable and easily practicable in the West. However, we are not sure if the self-treatment system was developed by Takata or if it too was part of what Dr. Hayashi developed."[43]

In terms of the initiation rituals, it appears that Mrs. Takata did not make any more changes in the rituals that she had learned from Dr. Hayashi; instead, it seems that she continued them in the form that she had learned from him. At least, this is the conclusion reached by Fran Brown, a Reiki Master initiated by Takata, who researched this issue many years later:

"I've worked with some of Hayashi's students/masters and they are delighted to find that my initiations and teachings of Reiki are the same as theirs."[44]

Jikiden Reiki

The Hayashi Reiki Manual was compiled by Frank Arjava Petter with Tadao Yamaguchi, the son of Chiyoko Yamaguchi, who had learned the Usui System with Dr. Hayashi at the end of the 1930s.[45] After Chiyoko Yamaguchi had taught Reiki "secretly" in Japan for many decades, this development took an unexpected course at the end of the 1990s: At that time, according to Frank Arjava Petter, "Chiyoko Sensei's son, Tadao Yamaguchi, attended a seminar about healing arts, at which he exchanged business cards with another participant. The business card that he received had 'Reiki Master' printed on it.

Tadao was very surprised and told the other person that his mother had already been practicing Reiki for 60 years. The other seminar participant was visibly irritated and told Tadao about a book on Reiki that his teacher Toshitaka Mochizuki (one of my students) had written. Tadao established contact with Mr. Mochizuki, and the Yamaguchis became well-known overnight in the Japanese Reiki scene, which mainly consists of Japanese who practice the Western Reiki."[46]

In the summer of 2000, Frank Arjava Petter went to Kyoto and spent five days there with Chiyoko Yamaguchi and her son Tadao to learn the First and Second Reiki Degrees in the same manner, as Dr. Hayashi had taught it sixty years ago.[47] "Meeting Mrs. Yamaguchi and her family heralded a new era in Reiki for me," Frank Arjava Petter writes. "In the presence of Mrs. Yamaguchi I felt the spirit of Reiki being transmitted with extreme clarity. I found Reiki in every smile, in every reassuring word this humble lady uttered, in every little healing hint she gave. In the way she moves, in the way she talks in each moment of her life. (…) In the summer of 2002 my dream came true and I began the Reiki Master Training under the Yamaguchis. This was the completion of one full cycle in my life. I left Japan and am living now in Germany, returning to my roots."[48]

On August 19, 2003, Chiyoko Yamaguchi passed away in the circle of her family at the age of 82 years. Her son Tadao Yamaguchi continues her life's work today. In Japan and other countries, he teaches the form of the Usui System taught to him by his mother on the basis of her experiences with Dr. Hayashi, which is now called *Jikiden Reiki*. *Jikiden* means something like the "direct transmission," so the term *Jikiden Reiki* can be translated as "the direct transmission of Reiki."

Joint Meeting

I met with Frank Arjava Petter for the first time in the summer of 2003. We talked about Reiki, the planned *Reiki Magazin* readers' trip to Japan that Frank Arjava would be leading, and much more. We spent a pleasant, relaxed time together. One year later, in the summer of 2004, when I visited him again, I had the opportunity to have an extensive conversation with Tadao Yamaguchi, who was in Düsseldorf holding a course in *Jikiden Reiki* at that time. Walter Lübeck was also there, so the four of us, each from a different tradition of the Usui System, were able to talk about the common factors and differences in our practice of the Usui System—which was an interesting exchange.

Hiroshi Doi

Another Reiki Teacher who has recently received access to new information about the life and work of Mikao Usui is Hiroshi Doi. After he had spent many years learning more than 30 methods of healing, he discovered the Usui System of Reiki for himself and recognized "that Reiki includes everything and Reiki harmonizes everything within itself."[49] He first learned The Radiance Technique® from the Japanese Reiki Teacher Mieko Mitsui, as well as Osho Neo-Reiki.[50] Shortly thereafter, he discovered the *Usui Reiki Ryoho Gakkai* and was trained by Kimiko Koyama, its president at that time, in the "traditional Reiki method according to Usui Sensei".[51] In the following years, he learned additional forms of the "Western Reiki" (this is the name used in Japan for the forms of the Usui System that have developed within the Western cultural region in order to compare them with the traditional methods according to Usui). In addition, Hiroshi Doi studied with the Japanese Reiki Teacher Chiyoko Yamaguchi, whose teachings he in turn compared with the traditional method according to Usui.[52]

Hiroshi Doi is the author of the book *Modern Reiki Method for Healing*, which was published in Japan in 1998 and appeared in English in the year 2000.[53] He is the honorary advisor for the *Nihon Holistic Reiki Kyokai* (Japanese Society for Holistic Reiki) and the Reiki One Healing Association.[54] Even if he is not an official teacher of the *Usui Reiki Ryoho Gakkai*,[55] he has been a member of this society since 1993[56]; this means that he is in close contact with other members, as well as with the teachers of the *Usui Reiki Ryoho Gakkai*, which have extensive knowledge about the Reiki healing method at the time of Mikao Usui. On the basis of his numerous experiences with a great variety of Reiki systems, Hiroshi Doi combined the "Western and Japanese traditional methods" and developed a new method of practicing Reiki: *Gendai Reiki Ho*.[57]

Gendai Reiki Ho

Hiroshi Doi writes the following about the development of this method: "In November 1993 I began to create the new method. After I had practiced it, tried it out, and definitively established its effectiveness a number of times, I worked out the entire system in October of 1996. In January 1997, I began imparting *Gendai Reiki-hô* to some of the naturopaths in Japan. Since then, about 2,000 people have participated in my seminars to date."[58]

Gendai Reiki Ho, according to Doi, is "a new method of practicing Reiki that is useful for modern people. The two main points of this method are: 'healing the soul and the body' and 'spiritual development.' The method is based upon the unification of the high spirituality of the traditional Reiki method (such as the teachings of Usui Sensei and the purity of the system) and the rationality of the Western method (the effective system that is accessible to everyone). The goal of this method is to make life peaceful and fruitful through simple everyday practice."[59]

The techniques of the *Gendai Reiki Ho* were developed on the basis of the following four starting points: "1. In examining the traditional and Western methods, 'healing the soul and the body' and 'spiritual development' are seen as the focal points. 2. Techniques are introduced whose effectiveness has been proved and established without any secrecy, belief in miracles, and mysticism. 3. Techniques are introduced that date back to the teachings and ideas of Usui Sensei and in which the qualities of Reiki unfold. 4. The techniques are simplified so that they can be easily used in everyday life."[60]

As Hiroshi Doi writes, Mikao Usui said "that Reiki is Ki (life energy) and simultaneously the light that fills the entire universe."[61] Furthermore, Doi states: "I am convinced that Reiki is the vibration of love, harmony, and healing from the universe. In order to receive this, it is necessary that a 'reception system' for Reiki be completed within us. The 'reception system' for Reiki means coming into harmony with the frequency of Reiki through self-cleansing and consciousness-raising. The techniques of the *Gendai Reiki-hô* are there to facilitate a resonance with Reiki. The 'reception system' is developed by consciously practicing the techniques every day. However, the goal is that we one day can constantly resonate with Reiki without being conscious of it and not that we optimally master the techniques to use them."[62]

Four Degrees

Gendai Reiki Ho, according to Hiroshi Doi, is "divided into four degrees that always involve how we resonate with Reiki and can increase the level of this resonance. The First Degree focuses on opening the channel through which the Reiki flows and learning the fundamental aspects of the Reiki treatment, which is based on resonating with the Reiki energy. In the Second Degree, three symbols are given for increasing the healing ability by resonating with the higher order of Reiki. In the Third Degree, the Master

Symbol is given and the goal is to achieve the first level of a state of inner peace and calm through practicing the techniques and exercises for spiritual development. The Fourth Degree involves deepening the practice for spiritual development and contributing to the spreading of Reiki and expanding the number of practitioners of love and harmony."[63]

In the First, Second, and Third Degree, the participants "receive three initiations for each. They receive three symbols in the Second Degree and another symbol in the Third Degree. In the Fourth Degree, they receive an initiation for the unification of the four symbols for an improved balance of all the symbols."[64]

Those who have attained the Teacher Degree of *Gendai Reiki Ho* "are not subject to any restrictions. They are permitted to act freely, whether they would like to impart *Gendai Reiki-hô* or integrate it with their own methods."[65]

Practical Exercise

A part of the practice of *Gendai Reiki Ho,* according to Hiroko Kasahara, one of its teachers, is the breath exercise on page 170; it comes from the Shintoism of ancient times and serves the cleansing of karma. A central element of the exercise is the Hado Breathing Technique. *Hado* means vibration. The Hado (vibrational) Breathing Technique, according to Hiroko Kasahara, has the same effects as other abdominal breathing techniques: stimulating the functions of the inner organs; increasing the absorption of oxygen; improving the metabolism, autonomic nervous system, hormonal secretion, and the immune system; increasing the active energy; deep relaxation; psychic stability; and more. In addition, because of its fine frequency this breathing technique has the effect of activating the chakras and increasing the consciousness vibration.

Seminars

Hiroshi Doi states that he basically organizes seminars once a month in Ashiya, Japan. "Seminars for the First and Second Degree only take place in Ashiya, which means that I do not organize seminars for these two degrees in other cities since I think that the students for these levels also need the support of their Reiki Master/Teacher time and again, even after participating in a seminar. When I receive inquires from distant places in Japan, I normally refer that respective person to a Reiki Master/Teacher in their own area."[66]

"For Reiki Teachers who have learned Reiki from another Reiki Teacher," Doi writes, "I organize special courses for Reiki Teachers in Ashiya and Tokyo. Outside of Japan, I organize these special courses within the scope of an URRI event after the workshop (this is the annual event of the *Usui Reiki Ryoho International* / see pg. 312, author's note). (...) This special course is oriented to those who are already Reiki Teachers in the Western methods. This two-day course focuses on understanding the spirit of Usui Sensei and the original essence of the Reiki method and learning what the First to Fourth Degree of the *Gendai Reiki-hô* involves from the standpoint of a Reiki practitioner, as well as from that of a Reiki Teacher."[67]

The energy-transmission lineage of the *Gendai Reiki Ho* is: Mikao Usui—Kanichi Taketomi (President of the *Usui Reiki Ryoho Gakkai* from about 1935-1960)—Kimiko Koyama (President of the *Usui Reiki Ryoho Gakkai* from about 1975-1999)—Hiroshi Doi.[68]

About Symbols

According to Hiroshi Doi, "symbols are shapes such as marks and letters and are considered as 'the antenna to tune into the universal energy.' Energy comes from some shapes or the waves resonant with

Cleansing the Spinal Column through Breathing
According to Hiroshi Doi, as instructed by Hiroko Kasahara

The goal of Gendai Reiki Ho is to achieve imperturbable inner peace by living in harmony with the universe. For our spiritual development and the achievement of this state, it is necessary to purify and dissolve our karma.

In the Shintoism of ancient times, it was said that God lives in the spinal column of human beings and all of the karma is recorded here. This is why it is necessary to cleanse the spine in order to completely purify the karma.

By practicing this exercise, the great life force that has gathered in the universe can flow through the spinal column. This can eliminate disorders in the spinal column and allow the cells of the entire body to become healthy. Since the techniques or exercises are not the actual goal in Gendai Reiki Ho but a means to coming into harmony with the universe, they will no longer be necessary when we have increased our spirituality.

1. Sit with a straight back. The eyes are closed.

2. Move the hands upward, above the head. Feel that the vibration of Reiki flows through the entire body like an internal and external shower, cleaning the body inside and outside. (Imagine a "Reiki shower" during the entire exercise.)

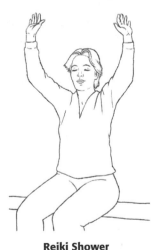

Reiki Shower

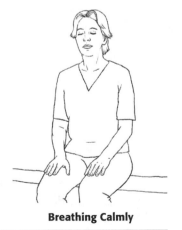

Breathing Calmly

3. Slowly bring the hands down to the thighs, palms facing downward. Keep the consciousness focused on the Tanden and breathe calmly. (The Tanden is the energy center located three fingerwidths beneath the navel.)

4. Hado Breathing Technique—Basics: Imagine the line from the Crown Chakra down to the coccyx (lowest part of the spinal column) as a pipe. Now slowly inhale and exhale using the Hado Breathing Technique. While exhaling, make a long-drawn, voiceless sound that comes from deep in the throat, similar to the breathing used when someone wants to warm cold hands. The tone created in this way, a voiceless "Haa" expressed through the breath is one of the original breath sounds of humanity, full of mystical power that resonates with the universal energy.

Hado Breathing Technique

5. Exhaling with the Hado Breathing Technique: While exhaling through the mouth, imagine that the hot steam of the breath is flowing from vertebra to vertebras, from above to below, and dissolves all of the dirt from the inside and outside of the pipe (from the Crown Chakra to the coccyx). You can also imagine that with each exhale a light laser-beam is dissolving all of the dirt from the inside and outside of the pipe. First let the breath flow from the top of the head to the coccyx, and then let it flow from there to the outside.

6. Inhaling: When inhaling through the nose, imagine that the divine pure water located in the sacrum is flowing upward through the inside of the pipe to the "third eye" (Sixth Chakra). (The sacrum is the lower bone of the spinal column that lies somewhat above the coccyx. In the Shintoism of ancient time, it was said that a pure, divine liquid is found in the sacrum. Today we know that there is a clear, colorless fluid found in the brain and spinal marrow.)

7. Repeat Points 5 and 6 a number of times. As you do this, count inhaling and exhaling for five times as one unit and do a total of three or five or seven units. Seven units are the maximum. Do not do this exercise more than once a day.

8. After the exercise, silently meditate for 5 to 15 minutes. With your eyes closed, keep your consciousness lightly focused on the third eye and breathe through the skin of the entire body. This will allow all of the cells to be filled with Reiki energy.

certain shapes (example—pyramids and spirals) and are known as the cosmic symbols which connect to the universal energy."[69]

At another point in his book, Hiroshi Doi explains his opinion on the topic of Reiki symbols: "The role of Reiki symbols is the same as supporting wheels of a bicycle when you try to ride it the first time. Anyone can ride a bicycle with supporting wheels. The shape of supporting wheels can be different as long as the 'supportive' function is satisfied. The same thing can be said of Reiki symbols. Symbols make the use of Reiki energy easier."[70]

According to Hiroshi Doi, Mikao Usui did not use any symbols himself, but Usui said: "Use symbols well. Use them more and more, and you will find yourself at the stage where you do not need symbols anymore. The human mind can reach any point in universe immediately. You need to grow so far that you do not need symbols anymore."[71]

About Dr. Hayashi

Further information about the formation period of the *Reiki Ryoho,* in this case about Dr. Hayashi, can be found in an interview with Hiroshi Doi by William Lee Rand, the publisher of the *Reiki News Magazine:* According to Doi, Dr. Hayashi was the last of Mikao Usui's students to be initiated by him into *Shinpiden,* the Third Degree.[72] From the very beginning, Dr. Hayashi had the support of Mikao Usui for his activities, including the establishment of the Reiki clinic in Tokyo: "Usui Sensei assigned a task to Hayashi Sensei, who was a naval doctor, to open a Reiki clinic apart from the *Gakkai* activities, in order to study and promote the efficacy of *Reiki Ryoho* from a medical doctor's point of view."[73]

Dr. Hayashi's founding of a new society, the *Hayashi Reiki Kenkyukai* (cf. pg. 41) also occurred with the support of Mikao

Usui. Dr. Hayashi supposedly had already founded this society while he was still a member of the *Usui Reiki Ryoho Gakkai*. He left this society after Usui's death, probably as the result of differences of opinion between him and the president of the *Usui Reiki Ryoho Gakkai* at that time, Juzaburo Ushida. It appears that a policy allowing Dr. Hayashi to study freely in relation to the *Reiki Ryoho,* which had been established personally by Mikao Usui during his lifetime, was changed after Usui's death.[74]

Re-Importing the Usui System

Since the *Usui Reiki Ryoho Gakkai* had just been acting in secrecy since the 1940s (cf. pg. 39), the Usui System of Reiki in Japan only became accessible again to a larger number of people in the mid-1980s. This occurred because some of the Reiki Teachers who had learned new forms of the Usui System in the USA and Europe, or from so-called "independent Masters" (cf. Chapter 7), went to Japan and began to give Reiki courses there. Such a "detour through the West" does not appear unusual at all for people in Japan. For example, Frank Arjava Petter has discovered that "it is a well-known and somewhat-numerous fact of Japanese culture that techniques developed in Japan often need to be exported to the West and then reimported to become accepted by the Japanese people."[75]

Within this context, it is interesting to keep the following fact in mind: Not only in Japan but also the rest of the world, more than 90 percent of all people who practice the Usui System of Reiki have received their fundamental initiations through a lineage that goes back to Mrs. Takata. Even the Reiki Teachers who offer the meditation techniques that date back to Mikao Usui or the Japanese-influenced forms of the Usui System generally became familiar with the Usui System through a teacher whose initiation lineage came from Mrs. Takata.

Learning and Teaching

Many Reiki practitioners now ask the question: What significance does the new information about the life and work of Mikao Usui and Dr. Hayashi have for my personal practice of the Usui System? In addition, this question arises for Reiki Teachers: What significance does this information have for my teaching of the Usui System?

In recent years, I have discovered that the new information has given me a different, we could say an "adult" context within which I can now move with my practice and teaching of the Usui System. Perhaps it is also that the history of the Usui System, which I tell in the First Degree seminar has become more extensive and clear in some places (even if I still tell the legendary form of the history in the seminar). Moreover, I let myself become inspired in my own practice of the Usui System by the way in which Mikao Usui and Dr. Hayashi apparently gave Reiki treatments. However, the heart of my practice and teaching of the *Usui Shiki Ryoho* according to Mrs. Takata has not changed.

In a seminar with Don Alexander, I learned some of the meditation techniques that probably came from Mikao Usui and practiced them on a regular basis in the following time. However, I discovered for me personally that these techniques lead me into an energetic space that is not in resonance with the essence of what constitutes my personal practice and what I teach in my Reiki seminars. Consequently, I did not continue to practice these techniques, and I also did not feel the urge to pass them on to others. Yet, I would not have missed the opportunity of becoming acquainted with them and having practiced them for a while.

I think that anyone who would like to pass on to others the techniques dating back to Usui and/or the way in which he practiced

175

Reiki should answer the following questions honestly: 1. Can the teaching of these techniques and treatment methods be integrated into my "teaching system" in a meaningful and energetically appropriate way? 2. Have I practiced the corresponding techniques and types of treatments long enough on myself on a regular basis before I pass them on to others?

In response to the last question, Frank Arjava Petter states: "The incredible speed with which information is disseminated today has allowed many Reiki teachers to present material that they themselves have not yet fully understood. This is an unfortunate side of the great Reiki explosion. The Japanese Reiki techniques that I myself uncovered in Japan have fared similarly. We began to teach these techniques only after we ourselves had practiced them for over a year and a half. It is really only possible to pass on to others what we know well."[76]

7. New Paths

Further Developments

For the approximately 80 years in which the Usui System of Reiki has spread around the world, a picture has emerged that shows one thing above all else: change. And this applies not only in terms of the various forms that the Usui System has taken in the course of time but also with respect to the works of the hundreds of thousands of Reiki Masters and teachers throughout the world who understand themselves to be "independent Masters" of the Usui System. These "independent masters" do not feel that they belong to any specific form of the system. In view of the immense number of practicing and teaching "independent Masters," the question arises: How did this development happen?

During Mrs. Takata's lifetime, among the Masters that she initiated it was generally well-known that she was the only one who initiated others into the Master Degree; at this time, the Masters initiated by Takata only taught the First and Second Degree. It was only after Takata's death in 1981 that the question arose as to who would initiate further Masters from that time on. As Phyllis Furumoto said to me, Takata probably gave all the Masters who she initiated the permission to initiate two to three new Masters before their own deaths so that the teachings and practice of the Usui System would be preserved and their own legacy could be passed on to others, allowing it to be continued in this way.[1] However, the question remained as to who would generally assume the task of initiating additional Masters after Takata's death.

After Mrs. Takata passed away, two of the Masters who she initiated understood themselves to be her successor (cf. pg. 82). One of these two Masters was Takata's granddaughter Phyllis Furumoto.

177

As she said, she received the blessing of the majority of the Masters present at the meeting by 17 of the total of 22 of Takata's Masters who met in 1982 on the Hawaiian Islands to become the successor of Mrs. Takata and perform the Master initiations from then on.[2] Within this circle of Masters, Phyllis Furumoto, as the acknowledged successor of Hawayo Takata, remained the only one to initiate new Masters for many years. At the same time, other Masters initiated by Takata, including Dr. Barbara Ray, began to initiate additional Masters.[3]

As Phyllis Furumoto said, she initiated five or six Masters relatively soon after Hawayo Takata's death; however, these were people who Takata had already foreseen for the Master Degree. Consequently, she had just continued the work of Takata. A short time later, she initiated the first person who learned the Usui System from her from the start into the Master Degree. However, difficulties arose between her and the newly initiated Master so that she initially distanced herself from any more Master initiations. She then dedicated several years to her own continuing personal development before she initiated any more Masters.[4]

As Phyllis Furumoto also told me, she received a special seal from Takata that had belonged to Dr. Hayashi.[5] It has been said that the seal used by the Masters of The Reiki Alliance on the certificates they issue is adapted from the seal belonging to Phyllis Furumoto.

"Decontrolling" the Master Initiations

In spring 1988, at the annual conference of The Reiki Alliance, which took place in Germany, Phyllis Furumoto held a speech that was to have far-reaching effects. She spoke to the Masters present there and shared her thoughts that from now on she would no longer be the only person who could initiate the Masters.[6]

What Phyllis Furumoto wanted to express was that, from her perspective, there were a few Masters who were now ready to give the Master initiations. However, her statement was generally understood to mean that now every Master was entitled to initiate new Masters.[7] Consequently, a downright "avalanche" of Master initiations began: With good intentions, many Masters initiated new Masters, who very quickly initiated more Masters on their own. However, many people saw that due to a lack of experience "the integrity of the form and embodiment of the practice which can only come from years of disciplined practice was lost."[8]

As a result of this development, there were increasingly more "independent Masters" who no longer saw their practice and teaching of the Usui System in correlation with a specific form of the system. Many of them changed the teachings of the system, such as the number and type of initiations, the hand positions taught, and some of the basic assumptions with regard to how Reiki works. However, the predominant number of these Masters still consider the major aspects of their practice and teachings to be based on the *Usui Shiki Ryoho* System according to Mrs. Takata.[9]

Because of the acceleration in the sequence of initiations, the Master-student relationship received a completely new orientation for many of the "independent Masters." While a long-standing, committed relationship usually occurred between the Master and the student before a Master initiation was given during Takata's time, there were now courses that took place on one weekend in which the "Master Degree" could be attained. Sometimes there was no long-term, committed contact with the initiating Master before or after such a weekend.[10]

Reiki and Money

Another element of the *Usui Shiki Ryoho* that was subject to considerable change during the course of this development for many "independent Masters" was money. Since many felt that the prices for the First Degree and Second Degree seminars, as well as for the Master training/initiation, commonly demanded by the Masters of The Reiki Alliance were too high, they lowered theirs. This frequently occurred with the argument that everyone should be able to access the universal life energy and that it is not fair to exclude people with weak finances from this possibility. This was also often accompanied by the assumption that the earth needs as much healing as possible and that the more people that are initiated into the Usui System, the more quickly the earth can heal as a whole.[11]

Interestingly enough, very few people who made these types of changes investigated the background for the price structure set by the Masters who are members of The Reiki Alliance. After all, this price structure was based on the teachings of Mrs. Takata and a specific, fundamental concept that proves to be correct upon closer examination.

Initiations and Follow-Up Initiations

Because of the different qualities in initiations into the three degrees, some Reiki practitioners felt the necessity of repeating their trainings or having their initiations performed anew. There are many different opinions on the topic of "follow-up initiations" or, as some people say, "new initiations" among Reiki Teachers. For example, while some teachers perform a follow-up initiation or new initiation into the First Degree with people who have learned it from another teacher and now want to receive the Second Degree from them out of principle because of the frequently major differences in the trainings, others believe that this is not necessary: The individual path of the students should be respected and it does not matter how they learned the First Degree since this fundamentally represents an adequate basis for the further personal path with the Usui System of Reiki.

Walter Lübeck believes that "additional initiations essentially have the effect of a strengthener sometimes even of a trigger for overdue processes of cleansing and re-orientation."[12]

In addition to the traditional initiations that take place in person within the scope of a Reiki seminar, the so-called "distant initiations" are also offered. These are initiations that a Reiki Teacher performs—in his own words—without the physical presence of the person who is to receive this initiation. Even if it may be true that such a practice actually functions when performed by very experienced and spiritually highly developed Masters, this procedure does appear to be far removed from any of the traditional forms of teaching the Usui System that I believe that the majority of all Reiki Teachers agrees that this form of initiation has very little in common with the Usui System of Reiki.

Inner Peace

In view of the increasingly numerous differences in the teaching of the Usui System, it is certainly healing to also keep in mind the common grounds that all Reiki practitioners have with each other. So we can first determine that all practitioners of the system, no matter what form they practice, share with each other the ability to transmit the universal life energy by laying on hands. Furthermore, all practitioners have been qualified to do this through the initiations that a Reiki Master/Teacher has performed for them. This means that every practitioner is part of an initiation lineage that, when followed back far enough, ultimately leads to Mikao Usui.

Connecting with the Inner Peace

By Tanmaya Honervogt

You can do this meditation either sitting or lying down—for example in bed as soon as you wake up or before you go to sleep.

Sit up straight and relax, close your eyes and let your breath flow naturally in and out.

Now put your right hand under the left armpit and the left hand under the right armpit. Relax and direct your whole attention to the chest area in between.

Allow a feeling of peace to rise from the heart. Just relax and direct your attention to this feeling.

When you are centered here and relaxed, you automatically come in contact with your inner peace. The heart becomes calm and sends out harmonic vibrations that you experience as love and peace.

Remain for about ten to fifteen minutes in this position, enjoying this feeling.

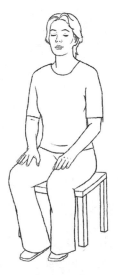
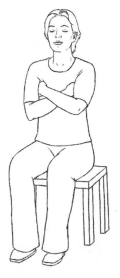

Breathe in and out   **Inner Peace**

Even if the various forms of the Usui System and the individual paths of the practitioners vary strongly from each other in some respects, they should—as far as they are practiced and lived in a responsible manner—ultimately lead to the same goal. Its essence is deep healing, inner peace, and universal love.

The exercise on page 182 with the topic of "Inner Peace" comes from the independent Reiki Master Tanmaya Honervogt and her book *The Power of Reiki. An Ancient Hands-on Healing Technique.*[13] I am happy that Tanmaya has contributed this exercise to the book.

Reiki in Combination

Many "independent Masters" use Reiki in combination with other methods of healing. Yet, many Masters who feel that they belong to a specific form of the Usui System in their teachings also combine Reiki with other methods of healing. General combinations are "Reiki and Bach Flowers," "Reiki and Aura-Soma," and "Reiki with Gemstones," for example. The chakra work with Reiki is also widespread. Another area is "Reiki and Sound."

As Walter Lübeck has discovered, "the legacy of Mikao Usui opens up a wide world of fantastic opportunities for healing and increasing the quality of life."[14] However, anyone who feels drawn to combining his or her Reiki work with other methods and systems should remember that it is advantageous to first learn to understand individual methods in their own essence and by themselves before combining them with each other.

Only when every healing method is experienced in its very own essence should the combination with different methods be attempted. Otherwise, a type of "energy mush" may occur in which the recipe or the mixture relationship is not totally harmonious. Instead of being more effective, the individual methods are then weakened in their effect or do not result in the correct overall picture. Anyone who treats himself/herself or others on a regular basis with a combination of various methods should do this on the basis of a responsible, knowing attitude. Once we have acquired an adequate understanding of each individual healing method that we want to use, then we can try combining the various methods with each other.

The following pages present an overview of the systems of Bach Flowers, Aura-Soma, gemstone work, the chakra teachings, and sound therapy. In addition, there is valuable information about how an experienced practitioner can combine these methods of healing with Reiki.

Bach Flowers

The following text gives an overview of the development and effect of the Bach Flower system[15]:

Bach Flowers are named after the founder of this natural method of healing: Dr. Edward Bach (1886–1936). He worked in London as a bacteriologist and homeopath before he moved to Wales in 1930 to dedicate himself completely to the development of this gentle system of healing. Even before this time, he had already had his own experiences with the enormous self-healing powers of human beings: he had suffered from cancer of the spleen in 1917 and, despite the poor prospects of healing, had become perfectly healthy again. Now he wanted to create a simple system of healing that anyone could use for self-treatment without risk. Using intuitive work over a period of eight years, he developed a system that included a total of 38 flower essences. The flowers come from plants and trees that grow wild and are prepared in a way similar to homeopathy. Bach discovered the healing effect of the various essences by trying them out on himself. When he died in 1936, he left his life's work to some of his long-standing, trusted coworkers. They established the Dr. Edward Bach Centre in Mount Vernon, Oxfordshire, Great Britain, where the spiritual legacy of Bach has been preserved to this day.

The causes of a disease, Edward Bach discovered, always lie in the emotional area. According to Bach, disease is neither cruelty nor punishment but solely a corrective measure; a tool that our soul uses to point out our errors to us in order to keep us from even greater mistakes, to prevent us from causing even more harm, and to bring us back to the path of the truth and the light from which we should have never strayed.[16]

Bach differentiated between 38 illness-causing emotional states, which he then divided into seven groups. These are: "fear," "uncertainty," "insufficient interest in present circumstances," "loneliness," "over-sensitivity to influences and ideas," "despondency or despair," as well as "over-care for welfare of others." Bach compared these illness-causing moods with the virtues of our higher nature, among which he included wisdom, strength, gentleness, and joy. Taking the respectively appropriate flower essence should help people develop the missing positive characteristics and/or virtues. For example, the flower essence No. 14 Heather is intended for people who suffer from loneliness, especially for those who get unhappy being alone for any length of time, always seek the companionship and find it necessary to discuss their affairs with others, no matter whom it may be. The positive characteristics to be developed in this case are sensitivity and a willingness to help others. In addition, these people need to develop a sense of security.

All of the 38 Bach Flowers are suitable for treating chronic diseases, as well as for the treatment of acute states such as situations of psychological stress. There are no known side-effects. Bach Flowers are very compatible with other naturopathic therapies, as well as

Reiki with a Bach Flower Essence
By Anita Bind-Klinger

1. For Self-Treatment:

Mindfully prepare the space or the framework in which you want to give yourself Reiki (an atmosphere with as little disturbance as possible, have the Bach Flower essence ready). You can select the Bach Flower essence that has already accompanied you for a certain time in a personal process or select an essence that now acutely comes to mind ("intuitively calls you").

Take a drop from the original tincture of the selected Bach Flower essence (the so-called stock bottle, which is the little bottle that contains the respective essence) and sprinkle it on your Third Eye—the point on your forehead between the eyebrows, also called the Forehead Chakra or the sixth energy center.

Attune yourself to Reiki in the customary way and place your hands on your face and forehead (1st basic position on the head). After a while, place them in the temple position and continue in the sequence as accustomed.

2. For the Treatment of Another Person:

Mindfully prepare the space or the framework in which you want to give someone Reiki. Set up the Bach Flower essence that the person to be treated has requested or that has already accompanied the individual for a while.

Take a drop of the Bach Flower Essence on your middle finger, then gently sprinkle and lightly circle the Third Eye of the person to be treated. Then put 1-2 drops of the essence in one of your palms and rub it into both palms.

Attune yourself to Reiki in the customary way and begin the normal procedure of a basic treatment (head, front of the body, and back positions).

Trust that the essence of the message will penetrate into the levels of the personality through the subtle bodies—Reiki flows without any wishes or desires. The result is opening, release, integration, or whatever is permitted to happen. The universal, intelligent life energy alone knows in connection with the healing forces of the flower essences where and how much or how deeply into which layers it can or should flow.

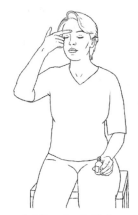

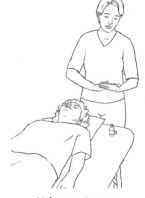

Sprinkling the "Third Eye"   **Using an Essence**

Additional Steps for Reiki II Initiates:

Reiki II initiates can send the message of the selected Bach Flower Essence during the mental treatment. The Bach Flowers represent certain life principles that are described in my book (as well as in other books) on Bach Flowers. Pay attention here to positively formulated wording. For example: If the Star of Bethlehem is used as

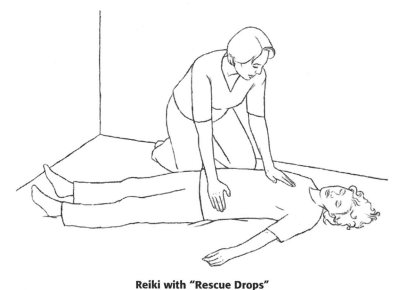

Reiki with "Rescue Drops"

the consolation flower, the message here could be: "I trust and grow in my life situations"—or for Impatiens as the flower of time: "Serenity and patience"—or for Holly, the heart-opening flower: "I open my heart and connect with the divine love in me."

Special Case: Reiki Treatment in an Emergency Situation

It is advised here to sprinkle the Rescue Remedy into the hands before the treatment with Reiki and let yourself be led in the situation as to where and how long the hands should touch the body.

with forms of conventional medical therapies; as a result, they are frequently used as an accompanying therapy. Even when they are taken in a "wrong" way (because of a mistaken diagnosis or overdosage) there is no risk whatsoever. For this reason, as well as the simple application of the system, Bach Flowers are very suitable for self-treatment.

However, one problem of self-treatment—whether with Bach Flowers or other easily comprehended methods of healing—is the "blindness to oneself" and the frequently lacking honesty toward oneself. It is not often easy to recognize what is lacking and it is all too human to not want to admit our own errors. Consequently, it becomes difficult to find the appropriate remedy. One possibility for dealing with this is making the selection of the flowers to be used in an intuitive manner. A set of Bach Flower cards can be helpful, for example. Those who have a complete set of the Bach Flower Essences at home can also directly select the bottles in an intuitive way.

The effects of the Bach Flowers lie on the subtle level. As in homeopathy, the healing power of the essences does not come directly from the physically detectable extracts but works through the energetic information contained in the flower, which is transmitted to the essence. The Bach Flower Essences are usually made in the following way: The flowers are first gathered at the peak of the blossoming period in certain places. Then they are placed in spring water and put out into the sun for several hours; this is how the vibrational energy of the flowers is transferred to the water. Finally, the derived water is poured into a sterile bottle and preserved in a specific mixing ratio with alcohol—then the storage bottles, the so-called "stock bottles" are ready.

Bach called his flowers the "cheerful dispositions of the plant world." Because of their energetic aura, they are capable of flooding negative emotional states with higher harmonious vibrations.

Since the 1970s, the Bach Flowers have found increasingly more supporters in Europe and the USA. Bach Flower Essences are available at health-food stores, either as a complete set or in single bottles. There are different ways to take the essences such as placing a few drops directly from the bottle on the tongue or mixing a few drops with some water to drink. In addition, the essences can be mixed in with creams, ointments, and body oils. Probably the best-known Bach Flower Essence is a combination of five different flowers, the so-called Rescue Remedy; this can be used for emotional stress and shock situations.

Dr. Edward Bach was not the only person who knew how to use the healing effects of flowers. Since ancient times, flowers have been used for their healing effects by the Australian Aborigines, the ancient Egyptians, and other early cultures, for example. In the 15th Century, the German physician and nature-researcher Paracelsus treated his patients with the dew that he had collected from flowers. Dr. Edward Bach discovered the healing effects of English plants in the 1930s for the modern world. Others followed his example, including Ian White who discovered the healing effects of Australian plants and created the system of Bush Flower Essences.

In the exercise on page 186, Anita Bind-Klinger, Reiki Master of the *Usui Shiki Ryoho* and author of the German-language book *Aura-Soma, Bach-Blueten und Reiki* [17], gives instructions on the use of Reiki in combination with Bach Flowers.

Aura-Soma

The following text provides an overview of the history, components, and effects of the Aura-Soma system[18]:

Aura-Soma is a holistic healing process that was founded by the Englishwoman Vicky Wall. She was the youngest daughter of a Cabbala master, the "seventh child of a seventh child" and had a close relationship with her father, who taught his daughter spirituality from a young age on. During her life, Vicky Wall was clairvoyant and could see people's auras. She worked as a pharmacy employee, chiropodist, and herbalist until, at an advanced age, she was led to the Aura-Soma system through a series of repeating visions within her meditations. In 1984, the 66-year-old Vicky Wall, who had now become blind, received the first recipes for the Aura-Soma Essences from the spiritual world.

A short time later, she met Mike Booth. After her death in 1991, he took over leadership of Aura-Soma as the Director of Production and Training. At the time of his first meeting with Vicky Wall, Mike Booth had worked as a management trainer. He immediately comprehended the significance of this new system, changed his future plans, and dedicated himself to the development of Aura-Soma from that time on. He worked closely with Vicky Wall and she trained him in how to make Aura-Soma Essences. Even today, he is still receiving new recipes for the Aura-Soma Essences in a clairvoyant manner.

The Aura-Soma system fundamentally consists of colored, fragrant oils and essences that are made of plant extracts and gemstone energies. By applying them to the skin or fanning them into the aura, the energies contained in the essences are sent to the corresponding areas within the energy fields of the body. Above all, the goal of using the Aura-Soma Essences is to develop energetic protection, strengthen the intuition, and support the healing processes.

191

The Aura-Soma system essentially consists of three product series: the Equilibrium Oils, the Pomanders, and the Quintessences. All of these products are colorful, fragrant substances in a variety of compositions and forms. There are more than 100 Equilibrium Oils, which represent the main series of Aura-Soma. These substances are contained in small, square glass bottles that each contain two different-colored liquids: the upper layer has an oil basis and the lower layer has a water basis so that the two do not mix with each other. The Pomanders and the Quintessences represent the two smaller series of Aura-Soma; there are about 15 of each respective series. These substances are made on a basis of alcohol. They are filled into small, convenient little plastic bottles that can easily be taken anywhere. All three of these product series are not limited, meaning that—at longer intervals—new essences are constantly added.

In order to become familiar with the Equilibrium Oils, it is important to speak with an Aura-Soma consultant who is trained to provide assistance during the selection of the bottles and the subsequent reading. The first Aura-Soma session generally takes place in the following way: You look at about 100 Equilibrium bottles that are all standing in rows on a shelf and then intuitively select four of them. In this process, the first bottle represents the personal mission in life ("the soul bottle"), the second one should throw light on current problems, blockages, and difficulties ("therapeutic bottle"), the third should say something about the path taken up to now ("mirror of the past"), and the fourth should reveal something about possible future perspectives. The four selected substances can be used in the time following the consultation.

It is also possible to use each of the 15 or so Pomanders and Quint-essences without previous instructions from an Aura-Soma consultant. While the Pomanders (bouquet of fragrances) are primarily intended to provide energetic protection, the Quintessences facilitate experiences with meditation and access to the archetypal images of the human psyche. Each Quintessence bears one or more names that were received by Vicky Wall in a clairvoyant manner; these come from the Theosophical teachings according to Helena Blavatsky, the ancient Greek world of the gods, various spiritual worlds, and the history of humanity. For example, the Quintessence No. 11 bears the names Lao-Tsu and Kwan-Yin; Lao-Tsu is considered to be a great wisdom teacher and the founder of Taoism, while Kwan-Yin is a female Buddhist deity who also represents the feminine yin principle. The use of the Quintessences is said to facilitate energetic contact with the corresponding Masters and an understanding of their work and messages.

There are extensive, summarizing lists for the three Aura-Soma product series that explain the ingredients and characteristics of the respective essence, as well as the therapeutic background. With the help of the lists, therapists who use other oils or even gemstones in addition to the Aura-Soma Essences can coordinate these with the contents of the essences used. The list for the Equilibrium Oils also contains classifications of the essences with the 78 Tarot cards of the Rider-Waite Tarot deck and the 64 hexagrams of the I-Ching. So the Equilibrium Oils can be also selected by using or taking into consideration these systems of wisdom, in addition to the intuitive methods.

The name Aura-Soma consists of the two individual words "aura" and "soma." In Latin, "aura" means "breath, vapor, shimmer"; it is generally used as the term for the subtle, electromagnetic field that surrounds the physical body. "Soma" means "body" in Greek and "lively energy" in Sanskrit. In this sense, there is no clear translation of the name Aura-Soma. One possible translation could be "the connection of the aura's energies with the body."

The products of Aura-Soma are available in many metaphysical bookstores or even directly from the Aura-Soma distributors on the

Reiki with an Aura-Soma Essence
By Anita Bind-Klinger

There are various essences by Aura-Soma. They are a bouquet of colors, fragrances, and gemstone energies. The Quintessences also contain a spiritual message.

1. Reiki Treatment with a Colored Aura-Soma Pomander

For Self-Treatment:

In as far as possible, select from the repertoire of the Pomanders to find the one that will be allowed to accompany you during the Reiki treatment.
Mindfully prepare the room or the framework in which you want to give yourself Reiki (an atmosphere with as little disturbance as possible, prepare the Pomander).
Put approximately two drops of the Pomander essence in your hands and rub it into your palms.
Attune yourself to Reiki, give thanks for the Reiki energy, and let the universal life energy flow free of wishes and desires in and out of you. As accustomed, begin with the first head position over the face and forehead. As you do this, consciously breathe in the fragrance of the essence. Continue with the positions in a sequence with which you are familiar.

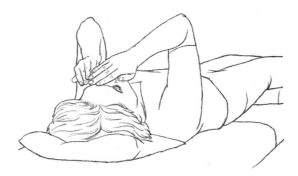

Consciously Breathing in the Fragrance

For the Treatment of Another Person:

If possible, the person receiving treatment should be able to select the Pomander for himself or herself.

Mindfully prepare the room or the framework in which you want to give someone Reiki. Set up the Aura-Soma Pomander that the person to be treated has desired or that has already accompanied the person for a while.
Put about two drops of the Pomander essence in your hands and rub it into the palms of your hands.
Attune yourself with Reiki in the customary way and begin with the first head position above the face and forehead with your hands that have been sprinkled with the Aura-Soma essence. Then continue in the familiar sequence of head, front of the body, and back positions.

2. Reiki Treatment with an Aura-Soma Quintessence

An approach similar to what has been described above applies here as well. You can select the Quintessence for self-treatment that has already accompanied you for a certain time—or it may intuitively call to you from the repertoire of the Quintessences at that moment. Before the Reiki treatment, sprinkle your hands with 1-2 drops and then begin with your customary self-treatment. Especially in the first position, consciously inhale the fragrance.

The Aura-Soma Quintessences contain spiritual messages that can be used in the mental treatment (for Reiki II initiates). For example: If the essence of Master Hilarion is used, the affirmation could be: "The way, the truth, the life." Or, for the essence of Lao-Tsu & Kwan Yin it could be: "I am connected with my deep wisdom and in loving compassion for all of Creation." The message when using the Holy Grail & Solar Logos could be: "Everything that I seek lies within me."

Whether in the treatment for yourself or for someone else, a Quintessence can also show up during a Reiki-Treatment (the name arises or something like that). In the subsequent time, this can be a meaningful and healing companion.

3. Reiki Treatment with an Aura-Soma Air Conditioner

All of the Pomanders and Quintessences are also available as Air Conditioners. Before the Reiki self-treatment, the selected essence can be included with a little squirt about 8 inches above the head.

Attention: These essences are very intense. A little squirt is enough, which will then slowly sink into the aura.

In the Reiki treatment for someone else, use a small (!) squirt about 20 inches above the head area and a little above the heart-solar plexus area. Then begin the treatment in the customary way.

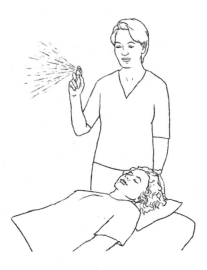

Little Squirt

Internet. Some of the essences are also available as Air Conditioner and the Pomanders can be purchased as creams, bath additives, etc. There are various advanced training courses in Aura-Soma throughout the world, including one by Mike Booth, the head of the Aura-Soma center "Dev Aura" in Tetford Lincolnshire, Great Britain. As the supporters of Aura-Soma like to emphasize, the essences are primarily suitable for an intuitively oriented, playful access to the spiritual worlds through the brightly colored and pleasant-smelling fragrances. There is a certain relationship between the Aura-Soma system and color therapy, as well as aromatherapy.

In the exercise on page 194, Anita Bind-Klinger, Reiki Master of the *Usui Shiki Ryoho* and author of the German-language book *Aura-Soma, Bach-Blueten und Reiki*[19] gives instructions on the use of Reiki in combination with the Aura-Soma Essences.

Gemstones

The following text provides an overview of the background and correlations in the healing work with gemstones[20]:

Gemstones are stones that have an outstanding position in the mineral kingdom because of special characteristics such as their beautiful coloring, their high degree of hardness, and their ability to polish well. Since the beginning of time, gemstones have been used in all of the known cultures as jewelry and for healing purposes: The stones are worn on the body as jewelry, talismans, or amulets; placed on the body's afflicted areas, for example, or ingested in a powdered form together with liquids. For example, in the ancient writings of Ayurveda there are precise instructions for preparing gemstone medicines in the form of elixirs, powders, and pastes. We know that the ancient Hebrews had gemstones decorating the jewelry of the kings and high priests. There were numerous different stones on the cuirass of the high priest to give him wisdom and protection, as well as healing qualities.

Beauty, rarity, and permanence—these are the three main characteristics that differentiate gemstones from the other minerals and make them into precious stones. Gemstones are tough, hard, and insensitive to outer influences, which is what makes them so durable. Their rarity also contributes to their value. And it is the task of the stone-cutters to bring out their beauty because they are usually found as raw roll pieces or in an impure form.

The healing effect of gemstones is based on the vibrations emanating from the stones. These vibrations arise from the crystalline structure of the respective stones, also called the crystal lattice, working together with light. The crystal lattice of a gemstone determines its physical, optical, and energetic characteristics. Overall, there are seven forms of crystal lattices: the cubic form, the tetragonal, the hexagonal, the trigonal, the orthorhombic, the monoclinal, and the triclinal. These result in the different forms of manifestation, colors, and energy patterns. At the same time, all of the gemstones that belong to the same crystal-lattice form have similar aspects in their energetic radiance. For example, gemstones with cubic structure have a very basic, earthy nature. Some people say that the energy that they radiate can contribute to the solution of difficult problems and for turning complicated ideas into reality.

Furthermore, the healing effect of gemstones is based upon the combination of the minerals that they contain.[21] In the course of their formation process, gemstones bind various minerals to themselves. The resulting, specific composition of the minerals plays a decisive role for the type of respective energetic radiation of the stones. The color of a gemstone is also determined by the composition of the minerals. The color effect of a stone also makes an important contribution to its healing effect.

In general, there is very little meaningful literature on healing work with gemstones. A standard work with concrete information on a total of 60 gemstones is the Lapidarius, created on the basis of extensive research by Marbod, the Bishop of Rennes who lived during the 11th Century. A short time later, the Christian mystic Hildegard of Bingen wrote her ever-popular works on subjects including knowledge on the healing effects of gemstones, which she had received through visionary revelations. Today's gemstone therapy is, as one of the specialized author points out, a mixture of traditions that have in part been assumed uncritically and hardly examined for their content of truth, channeled messages whose content cannot always be understood since they often relate to supposed applications during the age of Atlantis, as well as classifications with the planets and chakras, from which the special healing powers and spiritual effects of the stones are derived. In addition, there are observations by experienced practitioners who appear to be the only reliable source at this time.[22]

In addition to the ways of using gemstones for healing purposes already mentioned above, there are other possibilities for applying the energetic power of the stones in a spiritual manner. For example, gemstones are also used as meditation objects by holding them in the hands or having them serve as a visualization object. Fortune-tellers use crystal balls to catch a glimpse of the future, and healers employ gemstones to store energies and as supportive "tools" in working with the chakras (cf. pg. 206), for example. In this process, a specific gemstone that is energetically appropriate is moved in a circle above a chakra or up and down along the spinal column. Furthermore, gemstones can also serve as energetic protection and generally increase the personal life force.

Reiki Treatment with Quartz Crystal
By Ursula Klinger-Omenka

When Reiki is used in connection with gemstones, two great cosmic forces unite that stimulate each other in a very natural and simple way and develop a complex, reciprocal effect. The special quality of Reiki with gemstones is the natural and direct joining of both forces, which activates and increases them: and the result is more than just the sum of both energies.

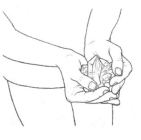

Quartz Crystal

Take a quartz crystal—in the form of a single, a small group, a tumbled stone (smoothly cut, simple stone), a pyramid, or a heart—and cleanse it under flowing water while you imagine how everything dark and burdensome is washed off of it. Then dry it with a clean towel, briefly hold it in your Reiki hands, and greet the crystal. Reiki activates its light forces on its own, but you can also imagine how the quartz crystal in your Reiki hands shines brightly in its pure light and glows like a big crystal of light.

Place the activated quartz crystal on the Heart Chakra, one of the other energy centers (chakras), or between the feet. Be sure that the stone is oriented in the optimal direction: The tip should always point upward to the head or point beyond the head if it is placed behind it. This stimulates an energy flow that leads to the "higher" potentials within us and opens up the optimal solutions—which also corresponds with the way that Reiki works.

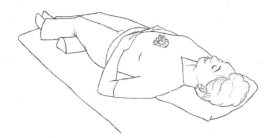

Self-Treatment with a Quartz Crystal

Now give the Reiki treatment to either yourself or a partner. When your hands touch one of the positioned quartz crystals while giving Reiki, you can simply place them on the stone. If it is a larger stone, place your hands around it. Reiki will then stimulate the crystal-light energy even more and flood this enormously intensified light force through the energy center where the stone and your Reiki hands are located, into the recipient.

Before you begin with the back treatment in the partner treatment, take the stone into your hands. After the person receiving Reiki has turned over, place it again. The best spot is the area of the coccyx so that the energy flows with intensification through the entire spinal column. After you have completed the Reiki treatment, take the quartz crystal back into your Reiki hands, thank it, and cleanse it in the same way as before the treatment.

An expansion and intensification is possible by placing seven quartz crystals during a Reiki treatment, one on each of the energy centers (chakras). In connection with Reiki, this develops a light-crystal bath and an extensive effective flooding of all the energy channels, energy bodies, energetic functions and processes on all levels of the person receiving Reiki with the cleansing, clarifying, organizing power of the quartz crystals.

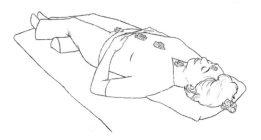

Self-Treatment with Seven Quartz Crystals

Please note: Before you give other people Reiki treatments in connection with quartz crystals or other gemstones, you should first have had experiences with using them on yourself by giving yourself a number of Reiki self-treatments with one or more quartz crystals.

In the quartz crystal, we encounter the manifestation of the pure light, a primal force of the Creation with which our soul forces feel connected. We "inwardly" long for this. This is also what flows to us with Reiki and works within us.

When a quartz crystal lies on the Heart Center during a Reiki treatment, the love and light in Reiki connects with the pure crystal light. United, this strong current of light flows into the innermost core of our Heart Center and merges with the flame of the eternal light within us. It allows it to become a lively, bubbling source of light, from whose abundance we draw clarity and pure love. In its flames, we are freed of any falsely understood (brotherly) love and purified. The unfolding cleansing, clarifying, organizing light forces strengthen us in being "pure hearted" instead of becoming engrossed in feelings but being "clear" with ourselves and others and acting from "pure" intentions.

We strengthen:

- Inner stability and focus with a quartz-crystal tip.
- How we live and work with others using a quartz-crystal group.
- The thankful recognition and acceptance of the mutual "polishing" and friction in the events of everyday life for our development with a quartz-crystal tumbled stone.
- The conscious connection with spiritual forces and their manifestation in the earthly realm, the mastering of the challenges of the material world with spiritual power and spirituality with a quartz-crystal pyramid.
- The pure love of the heart with a quartz-crystal heart.

The effect of placing seven quartz crystals is:

- Strongly supporting the clarity of our driving forces and our motivations in life in the first energy center.
- Activating the cleansing of the bloodstream and kidneys, promoting clarity in relationships and in creative processes in the second energy center.
- Dissolving blocked energy, anger, and annoyance; freeing the consciousness of self from exaggerated bossiness and self-control; and stimulating a natural simplicity in the self-image in the third energy center.
- Clarifying the expectation and disappointment in the love that we have in our hearts and developing pure love and joy of the heart in the fourth energy center (heart center).

– Strengthening clear communication that continually ensures clear circumstances, as well as the cleansing of the respiratory tract in the fifth energy center.

– Strengthening clarity of the imagination, in the ideas, and in the willpower in the sixth energy center.

– Stimulating a clear intuition that is free of egocentric perceptions in the seventh energy center.

The material value of a gemstone rarely reflects its value on the energetic level. For example, the diamond has the highest material value as the hardest of all gemstones but plays a rather unimportant role as a healing stone—it supposedly is put to the best use in connection with other stones in healing work. In addition, the diamond is considered to be a stone with a basic energy that increases the physical power of the person who wears a diamond ring, a diamond broach, or a diamond necklace. On the other hand, the heliotrope is not worth much in the material sense. However, in healing work it supposedly is excellently suited for producing the appropriate harmonization of the chakras. Seen in energetic terms, this also makes it a very important stone.

The healing effect of gemstones unfolds in a gentle and subtle way. Anyone who would honestly like to do healing work with gemstones is well advised to orient himself or herself upon the knowledge of an experienced practitioner. The more personal experience we have in the course of time, the more our personal knowledge about the "right" healing application of the stones and the more an intuitive approach to the stones will also be possible. For the initial experiences of energy work with gemstones, quartz crystal is very suitable because of its purity and clarity.

This applies to acquiring gemstones: If you are looking for high-quality stones, make contact with an expert or go to a good jewelry store. Gemstones can also sometimes be purchased for a fair price through stone-cutting workshops or specialty magazines. The connections between gemstones and other esoteric disciplines are frequently described. For example, there is an astrological gemstone theory that classifies each sign of the zodiac and every planet with one or more gemstone(s)—such as the amethyst with the sign of Pisces. Furthermore, there is a close relationship between the theory of gemstones and color therapy.

According to some of the esoteric sources, not all of the gemstones that exist on earth are equally significant for each era. There are even some gemstones that will only be important for human beings in the distant future. In addition, these sources also say that not every gemstone has a direct relationship to human beings.

⟝⟞

In the exercise on page 200, Ursula Klinger-Omenka, Reiki Master and author of the book *Reiki with Gemstones*[23], gives instructions for the use of Reiki in connection with quartz crystals.

She reports the following on the beginnings of her work with Reiki and gemstones: "When I received the First Degree in Reiki, I had the impression that this is enough! I felt that what had been triggered within me was adequate. And the same applied to the people to whom I gave Reiki: I did not have the impression that they needed or wanted more. The work with the stones then brought another intensity into my feeling for Reiki. I noticed that it is good to open myself to the Second Degree and continue on the path with Reiki. I have always experienced Reiki as the basis, as the foundation for what I am permitted to experience with the stones or even for what I would like to do with them. This has given me a sense of security."[24]

The Chakra Teachings

The following text presents a brief overview on the origins and background of the teachings of the chakras[25]:

The teachings on the chakras as energy centers in the subtle body of human beings is a component of many spiritual traditions. The various teachings generally recognize seven major chakras. These are located at the center of the body, along the spinal column and horizontally above each other. The seven major chakras form the "heart of the chakra teachings." Furthermore, there are numerous secondary chakras such as those in the palms of the hands and soles of the feet. According to ancient Hindu scriptures, there are about 88,000 chakras in the subtle body of the human being. When chakras are referred to in the following, this means the seven major chakras.

The word "chakra" comes from the Sanskrit and means "wheel." Clairvoyant people often perceive the chakras as "spinning disks of light" or as "energy vortexes." The chakras are frequently called "transformers for the cosmic life energy": They absorb the life energy that is present everywhere around us, transform it, and channel it to our subtle body. Through special exercises, the amount of energy that is absorbed and distributed in the subtle body can be heightened. Among other things, this results in an increase in the amount of energy and strength in the physical body. In addition, energy from the body is given back to the cosmos through the chakras. According to the teachings of Kundalini Yoga, the chakras are located on the level of the astral body.

The astral body is one of several subtle bodies that form the aura of a human being. (Examples of other subtle bodies are the etheric body and the mental body. The subtle bodies are invisible to the human eye, but clairvoyant people can see them. With the help of Kirlian photography, a person's aura can also be made visible.) The astral body, the seat of the chakras, possesses numerous energy channels through which the life energy flows. These channels are called Nadis. According to the ancient Hindu scriptures, there are about 72,000 of these Nadis.

The most important of all the Nadis, which is also the main energy channel in the astral body, is called *Sushumna*—in the physical body this corresponds with the spinal marrow in the spinal column. Six of the seven chakras are located directly on the *Sushumna*. The seventh chakra, the so-called Crown Chakra, is located on the crown of the head. In the Hindu scriptures, the seven chakras are each associated with a specific number of petals. The number of depicted petals correspond with the number of the respective energy channels that come from the chakra. For example, the fifth chakra, the so-called Throat Chakra is directly connected with the astral body with a total of sixteen energy channels.

Each of the seven chakras has its own name; these come from the Sanskrit language. Moreover, each chakra, with the exception of the Crown Chakra, has its own color and a mantra associated with it. For example, the fifth chakra, which is located in the throat area, is *Vishuddha*. Its color is sea-blue and its mantra is HAM.

People often speak of the Kundalini force in relation to the chakras. This is the resting cosmic force that lies in the lowest chakra, at the base of *Sushumna* located on the lower end of the spinal column. The Kundalini force is depicted on many illustrations as a coiled snake. It can be awakened through years of spiritual exercises such as yoga through the regular practice of breathing, body, and meditation exercises. Once awakened, it rises from the depths of the Root Chakra through all of the chakras up to the Crown Chakra. This creates different states of consciousness. If the Crown Chakra is reached, the practitioner supposedly goes into Samadhi, a state of spiritual concentration and collection. Still acting in the here-

and-now, from this point on he or she will continually remain in a state beyond time and space and causality.

In modern healing work, various forms of working with the chakras have developed. There are now many forms of energy work that include the chakras. Furthermore, there are various forms of free therapeutic and energetic work with the chakras that are not directly connected with other disciplines but see themselves as their own methods. The goal of this work is generally to dissolve blockages and negative energies in the chakras or to activate, open, or harmonize the chakras to make healing and spiritual development possible. One view is that the chakras are a connected system so that an energetic imbalance in one of the seven chakras has a negative effect on the energetic equilibrium of all of the chakras. In keeping with this, techniques for chakra harmonization or chakra-balancing are applied. In the different forms of free therapeutic and energetic work with the chakras, in addition to physical and breathing exercises, aromas, Aura-Soma essences, gemstones, sounds, colors, and various forms of meditation are also used.

Here is a brief keyword listing of the seven chakras as they are generally understood in modern esotericism:

1st Chakra: Root Chakra, Base Chakra—Color: red—Keywords: grounding, stability, primal trust, will to live, fundamental needs in life—represents the physical will to exist—located at the level of the coccyx, between the anus and the genitals.

2nd Chakra: Sacral Chakra, Abdominal Chakra—Color: orange— Keywords: sexuality, sensuality, creativity, physical pleasure, original feelings—represents the creative reproduction of existence—located above the top of the pubic hair.

3rd Chakra: Solar-Plexus Chakra—Color: yellow—Keywords: development of the personality, self-expression, determination, strength, power, abundance—represents the shaping of existence—located about one inch above the navel.

4th Chakra: Heart Chakra—Color: green—Keywords: love, compassion, healing, devotion, qualities of the heart—represents devotion to existence—located at the center of the chest.

5th Chakra: Throat Chakra—Color: light blue—Keywords: Ability to express, communication, openness, expansiveness—represents the expression of existence—located in the throat area.

6th Chakra: Forehead Chakra, Third Eye—Colors: indigo blue, violet—Keywords: intuition, mental powers, projection of the will, imagination, telepathy—represents realization of existence—located between the eyebrows and above the root of the nose.

7th Chakra: Crown Chakra—colors: violet, gold, white, or colorless—Keywords: spiritual growth, self-realization, universal consciousness, contact with the Higher Self—represents pure existence—located at the top of the head

Many specialized books list additional categories of classifications with the seven chakras such as healing remedies, fragrances, gemstones, metals, elements, symbols, planets, Tarot cards, sounds, affirmations, etc. However, anyone who is inspired by these is well-advised to question the origin of the information presented. There are now such enormous differences in the various chakra teachings even with respect to the colors associated with the individual chakras. According to the original teachings of Kundalini Yoga, the color of the lowest chakra is yellow and not red, which corresponds with the modern esoteric approach. Because of the differences between the various chakra teachings, it is important to make sure that the individually used elements all come from the same teaching before using mantras or visualizations, for example.

Reiki and Chakra Work

The connection between Reiki and chakra work is widespread among Reiki practitioners, especially among the "independent Masters." Moreover, the direct energetic work with the chakras is a component of some forms that are based upon the Usui System such as *Rainbow Reiki, Rei-Ki Balancing®,* and *Osho Neo-Reiki* (cf. Chapter 5). On the other hand, the knowledge of the chakras is not a component of the teachings of the *Usui Shiki Ryoho* System headed by Phyllis Furumoto and Paul Mitchell. Mrs. Takata, according to Paul Mitchell, did not teach a direct treatment of the chakras.[26]

The work with the chakras, especially with the Heart Chakra, is the focus of various practical exercises contained in this book (such as "Feeling the Heart Space" by Himani H. Gerber, pg. 125, and "Chakra Development with the Reiki Powerball" by Walter Lübeck, pg. 108).

The most widespread form of working with the chakras among Reiki practitioners is the so-called chakra-balancing, which is sometimes also known as chakra-harmonizing. In this process, the seven major chakras are treated with Reiki one at a time, whereby the universal life energy is guided directly into the chakra. Various forms of chakra-balancing are well-known, such as the two following methods:

1. Treating each of the seven major chakras with both hands at the same time, for example from top to bottom (meaning that this form includes seven hand positions).

2. Treating two of the seven major chakras at the same time with one hand on each of them. For example: the Root Chakra and the Crown Chakra at the same time, then the Sacral Chakra and the Third Eye at the same time, then the Solar-Plexus Chakra and the Throat Chakra at the same time, and finally the Heart Chakra with two hands at the same time (meaning that this form includes four hand positions).

The World of Sound

The following text presents an overview of the origins and forms of healing work with sound[27]:

Since the beginning of time, sound has been used by human beings for healing purposes. In the early tribal cultures, the shamans used monotone, repetitive chants that are frequently accompanied by steady drum rhythms. This creates trance states that are intended to facilitate the transition into other states of consciousness. These types of practices are still a component of shamanic rituals today.

The *Upanishads,* the ancient Indian spiritual teachings, speak of a primal sound of the Creation, of *Nada.* All other sounds are derived from this primal sound, according to the *Upanishads.* In turn, the Sanskrit alphabet with its 50 letters, meaning the entire Sanskrit language, has developed out of this variety of sounds. Seen in this way, the things were not in the world first and then given names, but sound is what created the material world in the first place. A similar perspective is also expressed in the familiar Bible verse "In the beginning was the Word." The same applies to the Creation myths of many indigenous peoples such as the Aborigines whose "Songlines" say that the world was sung into life through sound.

The *Upanishads* state that:

> "The essence of all beings is the earth,
> The essence of the earth is the water,
> The essence of the water is the plants,
> The essence of the plants is the human being,
> The essence of the human being is speech,
> The essence of speech is sacred knowledge,
> The essence of sacred knowledge is the word and sound,
> The essence of the word and sound is OM."[28]

211

As Joachim-Ernst Berendt established in his book *Nada Brahma. The World is Sound,* the entire world, including everything in it and even the entire cosmos, is actually constantly creating tones. Plants create tones when they grow. Planets create tones on their path through space. Even if we as human beings cannot directly hear most of these tones since they are at a frequency inaccessible to our hearing, these "inaudible" tones have an effect on us.

In addition to these "inaudible" sounds that surround us everywhere, there are many other, audible sounds around us every day. The healing work with sounds involves creating those sounds that serve our healing and avoiding those that stand in the way of our healing.

Some of the classical instruments are especially well-suited for healing music such as the flute and the guitar, or the sitar, an Indian plucked instrument. Even modern synthesizers can create healing sounds—for example, the Indian Master Sri Ganapathi Sachchidanda Swamiji gives healing concerts on synthesizers accompanied by classical instruments. Natural instruments such as the didgeridoo—the large, long musical instrument carved from wood by the Aborigines—create healing sounds. The earthy sounding tones of the didgeridoo with their "wah-wah effect" go to the bone.

Special instruments that are used in the healing work with sound are the so-called overtone instruments. These create overtone music in which the relationship between each individual tone with a multitude of other tones is strongly emphasized and felt. Peter Stein, an instrument-builder and sound expert explains this in the following manner:

"Whenever a tone sounds, we hear a complete sound in reality. This consists of fundamental notes that determine the pitch and countless additional tones that are somewhat quieter as they resonate through the fundamental note and form the tonal colors—the overtones. The physical properties of an instrument determine which tones of the overtone spectrum are louder, which ones are quieter, and which ones do not resonate at all. Overtone instruments are instruments that can be played even without any previous knowledge because of their simple construction, making it possible to meditatively focus on the sound itself. Already thousands of years ago, such instruments were used in different ways for healing."[29]

A special form of overtone music is overtone-singing. This is a vocal technique that forms as many overtones as possible. Overtone-singing is a meditative variation of singing that dates back many centuries. It is a component of the religious rituals in numerous Eastern cultures such as those in Tibet, India, Japan, China, and Siberia. In addition to the extraordinary sound effect that overtone-singing has on the listener, it primarily imparts a sense of inner peace and security, which gives it a healing effect.

In terms of the effects of sounds on human beings, we can differentiate between two different types of effects. On the one hand, we perceive sounds through the ears. As we do this, the sound waves are transformed into nerve impulses. This is how they reach the brain, where they trigger moods, for example. On the other hand, the sounds directly affect the physical body. The sound waves travel through the body because of the high water content there and cause the tissue to vibrate. One form of sound work that is primarily based on this second principle is sound-bowl massage.

What is probably the best-known form of healing sound work is based on the ancient knowledge of the effect of sounds, which was already applied more than 5,000 years ago in the Indian healing arts. The singing-bowl massage uses singing-bowls rich in overtones (such as the Tibetan or Indian). The different sizes of bowls consist of various metal alloys and are similar in their form to essence bowls.

They are usually used on the body of a person in a supine position at the level of the chakras, for example. Then they are tapped with a striker or wooden stick and the sound is created by rubbing it along the edge of the bowl. According to their size and weight, the singing-bowls create different tones that reverberate for a very long time. Humming, singing, and hovering sounds are created. The vibrations are transferred to the body, making it possible to release tensions and blockages. In its modern form, the singing-bowl massage was developed by the German Peter Hess.

As the Indian teacher Krishnamurti already discovered, it is not just the ears with which we perceive sounds. Instead, every form of sound effecting human beings is a holistic process:

"We hear not only with our ears but also we are sensitive to the tones, the voice, to the implication of words, to hear without interference, to capture instantly the depth of a sound. Sound plays an extraordinary part in our lives: the sound of thunder, a flute playing in the distance, the unheard sound of the universe; the sound of silence, the sound of one's own heart beating; the sound of a bird and the noise of a man walking on the pavement; the waterfall. The universe is filled with sound. This sound has its own silence; all living things are involved in this sound of silence. To be attentive is to hear this silence and move with it."[30]

Reiki and Sound

How can Reiki and sound work be connected? Regarding one type of combination, all Reiki practitioners are experts in a certain sense: Almost everyone uses accompanying music more or less frequently during treatments with Reiki. Therefore, the music becomes a component of the treatment and has an effect on the person receiving treatment, in addition to the Reiki. It is important to select the respectively appropriate music to support the healing process in

Reiki, Sound, and Gratitude

By Dagmar Fröhlich

You will need the following for this exercise:
– A blanket or a yoga mat
– A small pillow
– Some water to drink

Go to a place with flowing water such as a small stream or at the ocean where you can easily hear the natural sound of the water and feel safe and secure. If it is hard for you to be alone in nature, ask a friend to accompany you and do the exercise together with you or just be close to you while you do it. Perhaps you can have a picnic together afterward.

Sit down, spread your blanket, and get comfortable. Take the time to watch and listen to the music of the water in its liveliness.

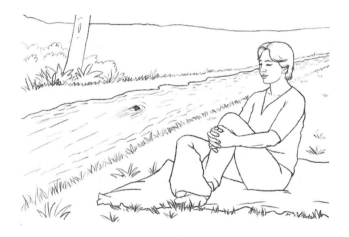

Listening to the Water

Become aware that this lively gurgling and babbling—usually inaudible to your ears—also exists within you. Your body consists of more than 70 percent water. Your relationship with the element of water is something very archaic. Even before your birth, you spent about nine months being surrounded by the element of water (in the form of amniotic fluid). Even at the four-and-a-half month point of the pregnancy, your ears were

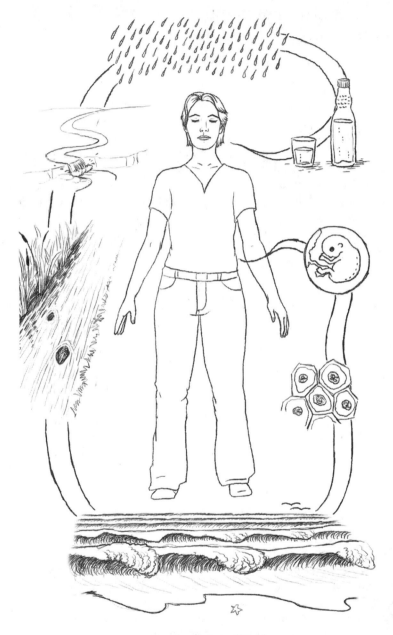

The Circulation of Water

completely formed and your original hearing experience began in the water. So the sound of water is very familiar to you. Water is very good conductor of all types of sounds. Since your body consists of more than 70 percent water, the absorption of all types of sounds, including the sounds of the water and of words, into your cells is supported.

Be certain that every good, pleasant-sounding word has positive effects on the structure of your body's waters, even down into your cells.

Now remember the fifth Principle: "Show gratitude for every living thing." The word "gratitude" is a very powerful word. When you give yourself Reiki right here near the water, let a mental "thank you" flow into every Reiki position that you use. Support this through your breath in the following way:

Inhale "thank you." During the exhale, guide your mental "thank you" with the flow of your breath to exactly where your hands are located on the body. As if on its own, your "thank you" will unfold there and have a positive effect. Your body, as the "temple of your soul," will thank you for it.

Now lay down in order to give yourself Reiki. If you are next to a stream, position yourself with your body in the direction of the stream's course: as if the stream was running from top to bottom, from your head to

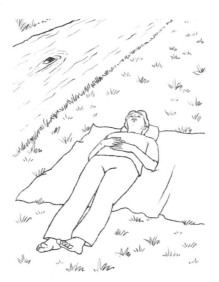

Self-Healing at the Water

your feet as it flows through you. If you are at the ocean, lay down at a respectful distance from the waves with your feet in the direction of the water. Remember that the water "wanders" because of the tides and take this into consideration when choosing a place to lie down. Now close your eyes and just listen to it.

After a while, attune yourself to receiving Reiki.

Then begin giving yourself Reiki. Treat the front side of your body. Begin at the head, with your eyes. Wait until Reiki is flowing well. First let your "thank you" mentally flow into you in this position. Inhale "thank you." During the exhale, direct your "thank you" with the flow of your breath to the eye area where your hands are now placed. As if on its own, your "thank you" will unfold and have its effect there.

Before you change to the second head position, simply give yourself Reiki and continue to listen to the sounds of the stream or the ocean. Use the same approach for the second head position and for all of the following positions. You can be certain: Your body will very gratefully accept the sound of the words "thank you" and the Reiki energy.

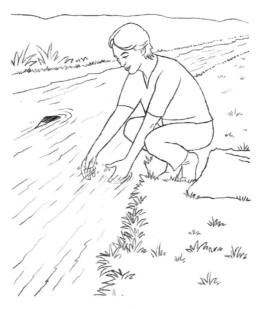

Thanking the Water

Continue to listen to the sounds of the water and enjoy them. Gradually complete the Reiki treatment. Open your eyes and slowly come back into the here-and-now.

Then go directly to the water and hold your hands into it for a short time. Give the stream or the ocean Reiki and thank it as a life-giving and preserving element for its wonderful sound. Also enrich the drinking water that you have brought with you for a few minutes with Reiki, then drink and simply enjoy it. Be conscious of how much good you can do for yourself and also for the natural world with Reiki, as well as how lively the Reiki Principles are, especially today.

the best-possible way. Accompanying music is sometimes also used as an external wall of sound to drown out noise from the street, for example, with the goal of creating a more healing atmosphere. However, we should not forget that it is also interesting to do treatments in silence and/or simply integrate the already existing background noise and not feel that it is bothersome.

A special form of sound work in relation to the Usui System of Reiki is chanting the so-called *Kotodamas*. The name of each of the three symbols of the Second Degree, as well as that of the so-called Master Symbol, can be used to create a corresponding *Kotodama*. According to Don Alexander, the chanting of such *Kotodamas* during Mikao Usui's lifetime was a common practice (see pg. 33). A *Kotodama*, within the context of the Usui System, is the tonal essence of the respective symbols, for the most part reduced to the vowels of its name. It serves the practice of chanting, which is repeated singing on one pitch.[31]

There is no agreement within the Reiki scene as to whether or not the complete names of the three symbols of the Second Degree and the so-called Master Symbol can be called mantras on their own. The answer to this question is ultimately dependent upon the definition of the word "mantra." Using a broad definition, every word can more or less be called a mantra if it is thought or sung as a meditation help. Seen in this way, the names of the symbols can also serve as mantras. A narrower definition, which is closer to the original meaning of the word, indicates that a mantra is a "mysterious, magical word" that is thought or sung as a meditation help. With this perspective, only specific words that are charged with magical power can be called mantras. Many people are convinced that this does not apply to the names of the three symbols of the Second Degree or the name of the so-called Master Symbol. For example, Phyllis Furumoto and Paul Mitchell expressed the opinion at an event in October 2002 in Gersfeld, Germany, that the names of the symbols are not mantras. Frank Arjava Petter has written the following on this topic: "In Japanese Reiki system of Dr. Mikao Usui and Dr. Chujiro Hayashi, the Mantras of the power symbol and the mental-healing symbol are not spoken out loud. They are simply regarded as the names of the symbols."[32]

One practice of the Usui System in which a tonal effect played a role that was customary during the period of Usui and Hayashi was reciting the Reiki Principles (see pg. 21). According to the tradition, the Principles were recited together at the meetings and in the courses, and the practitioners were admonished to "recite the five principles mornings and evenings while meditatively sitting still in the *Gassho* posture and to mentally repeat them, cultivating a pure and healthy mind as a result and translating the five principles into action in everyday life."[33]

Oral Tradition

Sound and/or the sound of words are also an essential aspect of one of the nine elements of the form of *Usui Shiki Ryoho* according to Mrs. Takata: the Oral Tradition (cf. pg. 93). Paul Mitchell writes the following on this topic:

"The essence of Oral Tradition can best be understood if we think of human experience before writing. (...) In pre-writing cultures, the most essential knowledge is transmitted person to person—learning what it means to be human, what life is about, its purpose, call, meaning, and how the world works. In this context, an energetic transfer occurs as the information is given, continuing an unbroken line of energy that connects through each ancestor to what has been learned, felt, lived by those who came before. This is the essence of Oral Tradition."[34]

Perhaps this is what is meant in the *Upanishads* (cf. pg. 211) when they say:

"The essence of the human being is speech,
The essence of speech is the sacred knowledge,
The essence of the sacred knowledge is the word and sound
(...)"[35]

Researching the Sounds

While some Reiki practitioners who perform the special forms of healing sound work, directly connecting it with the use of Reiki through methods such as a singing-bowl massage and giving Reiki just before, during, or after it or through additional chanting during a Reiki treatment (as is practiced in *Karuna Reiki®*, see pg. 135), other Reiki practitioners think it is important to not directly combine the use of Reiki with elements of healing sound work but instead perform them separate from each other. This second group of people includes the German Reiki Master and therapist Dagmar Fröhlich, who already has been exploring the world of sound for many years.

"For me," Dagmar Fröhlich writes, "both Reiki as well as the gift of the healing work with sounds has been and continues to be the result of an intensive personal, spiritual development with many ups and downs. It was and is worthwhile for me to have spent many years on this path and still be on it. I value and love both of them as a spiritual path and know that both come from a universal source. I also know that the one was born out of the other at the point in time when I was willing to open myself, in this case, to the sounds."[36]

"Even as it becomes an instrument of my highest consciousness," Dagmar Fröhlich says about her form of sound work, "I follow and trust its intuitive inspirations and play the singing bowls very individually for a particular person or the groups attending my concerts with the overtone sounds of the Tibetan. Supported by my inner, spiritual attitude of appreciation, uniqueness, and love, the vibrations of the sounds open those spaces of consciousness in the soul of the listener that need healing. In the individual therapeutic work, the sounds often come into resonance with the buried experiences of childhood, the prenatal phase, and those of other incarnations. Completely on their own, similar to what happens when we give Reiki, they bring up from the subconscious mind the theme that requires a step of resolution and integration in the life of the client precisely at that moment. In the process, they also dissolve physical blockages. In the form of the sound work that I have developed, the singing bowls are not placed on the body. Instead, I place them around the person in keeping with the experiences that I have had in body and energy work since 1989."[37]

"In the concerts," Dagmar Fröhlich continues, "the sounds strengthen the entire physical system, sweep the listeners into colorful worlds of images. They bring spiritual expansiveness and clarity, and much more. One thing that is especially fascinating about this: Born from the original source of all being and the harmony of the spheres, these meditative sounds touch our hearts and fill us with deep peace, reconciliation, joy, and gratitude in daily life."[38]

The exercise on the topic of "Reiki, Sound, and Gratitude" on page 215 was created by Dagmar Fröhlich for this book.[39]

8. Transcendence

Crossing the Borders

My way of practicing the Usui System is strongly characterized by spirituality. My personal approach to the Usui System of Reiki is based upon my wish for a simple spiritual practice that I can do on a regular basis. In the first years after my Initiation into the First Degree, I assumed that the form of the Usui System I practiced, *Usui Shiki Ryoho,* was a far-reaching spiritual discipline whose regular practice would make possible continuous spiritual development and transcendence[1]. However, after many years of practice I came to a point where I had to admit that this no longer applied for me.

I noticed that something was lacking for me in my tradition of the Usui System, *Usui Shiki Ryoho.* I could not really put my finger on exactly what this was at that time. In any case, I began to search for what I could not find in my tradition in the encounters with Reiki Masters who came from other traditions or had long left the boundaries of traditions far behind them. Through these personal encounters, I gradually found my way to something that I had believed was not there or would have to be searched for in the outside world and I recognized: It had been there the entire time within myself—I simply had not yet been able to access it.

Today, in addition to my regular practice of *Usui Shiki Ryoho,* various forms of meditation, as well as personal encounters with good Reiki friends and spiritual masters help me in finding this access anew time and again. In addition, I study various spiritual perspectives and philosophies, which help me develop an understanding and achieve lasting inner peace.

Reiki Master Meeting

A short time after my initiation into the Master Degree, I participated in a Reiki Master Meeting for the first time. It was held in Berlin. Sabine Fennell was also among the Masters present. I immediately felt a good connection with her. Sabine told the group that she had stopped holding Reiki seminars some time ago in order to concentrate completely on her work as a channeler and give channeling sessions. At that time, I tended to be critical about channeling. Yet, there was truth in what Sabine said and the energetic charisma that radiated from her set in motion processes within me that supported my spiritual development.

About one year later, I attended a channeling session that Sabine held. I perceived the tangible light-filled energy that was in the room and had some insights that let me understand the bigger picture. Our personal contact became deeper at additional meetings. I began to become more closely involved with the phenomenon of channeling.

The following text offers a brief overview on the background and correlations of channeling[2]:

What is Channeling?

During a channeling session, a psychic person, also called a medium, imparts information or messages to those who are listening or later reads a record of it. Sometimes the contents are also written down directly; however, this tends to be the exception. People usually come together in a group to a channeling session where a medium uses his or her voice to channel messages or information from spiritual sources to those present in the room.

A parapsychological perspective assumes that mediums receive the contents of their channeling through unconscious telepathy

Contact to the Spiritual Guides
Channeled by Sabine Fennell

Dear Reader of this Book,

We greet you from the heart. We, the oneness of Dr. Usui, who will speak to you first to let you know who we are and how we work in the spiritual realm through you, with you, and, above all, for you. We are so connected into your earth field that we optimally spin the threads, first in the spirit, and then also in a very real way, to once again produce more connections that are greater in number and more powerful than before, quicker and more flowing than before.

We have always been here and now are much better known under this name, much more than even just a short time ago on the earth. We have united as Dr. Usui to serve you now in a special way, dear reader, in this language and in this writing. This involves more healing, more completeness, and more perfection. You rise up in this field of happiness in a way that is increasingly brighter, faster, and smoother to give yourself energy and the absolute love of your heart. So know that you are not alone with your gifts on the earth. Instead, you are in an alliance with all Reiki people and above all, those who gather under this name time again to give conscious love to this field here on the earth and beyond, even into the cosmic field, into the totality.

We Usui-helpers are both Reiki-helpers and God-helpers at the same time. We give you everything that you need now in order to absolutely fulfill your own life plan so that it is easy for you to stand in life and simple for you to fulfill the programmed tasks that you have selected for yourselves. Seen in this way, we are also fulfillment-helpers and like to be in contact with all of you, in the case of Reiki through the gifts of energy that can be felt more or less but that increase with each Reiki gift of love so that you grow into abilities of all types. Bit by bit, you progress and increasingly enjoy your life, with more certainty in your heart: I am and remain healthy. I am and remain absolutely on my course in life in order to clearly and purely fulfill my life plan.

Above all, know that we Usui-helpers in the Reiki field give to you in a way that is very strong, very powerfully effective, and perceptible with all of the senses. So train all of your senses. Be open in meditations, above all to receive what is coming, through spirit, through God, and through us spiritual helpers of all types. Ultimately, you only need the open silence. When you are open and receptive in your hearts, it will be given to you in the best-possible way—always and everywhere. And if you favor meditations, you will notice how quickly you thrive now and progress with openings of all types that enable you to draw on more creative processes directly from your heart and offer them to the world as a gift.

Be an absolute gift yourself. Be happy that you are and remain in contact with spiritual guides in this simple way, consciously perceiving this more and more with all of your senses as well. Be clairaudient, clairvoyant, clairsentient, clairauditory, clair-tasting, and also be more telepathic as you move through the worlds. Simply greet everything and everyone with a loving, open heart, creating in this easy way a reconnection, a Religio, to everything that exists.

If time and again you cultivate this, meditation with a loving reconnection to everything that is, you will be a ray of sunshine on the earth. The sun in your heart will always shine absolutely, without stopping, without differentiating, on everyone and everything, for everyone and everything. This is always the goal of an awakened person, a fulfilled human life. And you are the one who ultimately defines anew the dimension of this bright sun, this bright power of the sunshine, refining it for yourself time and again in the here and now, training and checking yourself anew in a quiet minute and above all in the here and now. And then we spiritual helpers have special and absolute access to you and we also like to train you by speaking through you directly, as Sabine, the medium, is now speaking and also experiences anew time and again.

The mastery is naturally inherent within you. And yet, it wants to be opened again and radiate absolutely. Mastery in life means: I master my life. I am here in full presence, absolutely conscious of everything that happens within me and around me, and lovingly leaving everything there just as it is since it is as it is due to choice, for everyone and every-thing.

This is perfected mastery and it leads you into ecstasy and bliss without end—obviously with small exceptions since you are woven into the human field and will still stay for a good while, and in this way also participate and take part in everything that also happens in this earth field and resonates and flows through you and glows through you. So also accept the little stumbling blocks that occur time and again as part of the bargain. Even as a master, you are still here as a human being and should not completely lose the compassion that you have for your fellow human beings who you serve in the outside world and who also serve you at the same time.

So be in contact with God. Be in contact with Reiki. Be in contact with spiritual guidance, in a very concrete way that becomes increasingly tangible and distinct. We are always there, always available if you call on us, and we will give you exactly what you request, in addition to what you are carrying within as a possibility so that you open up more quickly and easily and live and love on the earth.

We are the oneness of Dr. Usui and would also like you to address us in this way, dear reader, so that you can simply embrace all Reiki people and beings in your mind, with this loving connecting track in your hearts, with this address, before you formulate a request or before you would simply like to communicate with us, in whatever way and for whatever purpose that may be. When you call upon us under the name Oneness of Dr. Usui, all of the Reiki forces are available to you in union and give to you powerfully in the here and now for healings, for conversations, even for all types of creative forms of expression, for everything that is on the agenda at the moment and for you.

Be certain that we very much like to resonate with you and give to Mother Earth with the highest power of love, which you also nurture, standing in alliance with all Reiki people, with all human beings who affirm, search, and find God in the silence more and more frequently, with growing ease, and increasingly smooth way.

Be loved. Be honored. And please absolutely honor this book here as a whole. Everyone who is participating here is also filled with spirit to the highest degree of his self and gives you the best, the finest, that he can present, especially to you at this moment.

Be absolutely loved. Be honored. And be in an alliance with all of us in the spiritual realm.

Amen.

or extrasensory perception from the unconscious minds of other people. Another theory expands this view even to the collective consciousness of humanity, which is also called the Akashic Records or world consciousness. According to this view, everything that has ever been said, done, thought, or felt can virtually be tapped into by sensitive people since everything is stored in the world consciousness that anyone has ever perceived or expressed. Seen in this way, the channeling material does not contain anything new—in any case, nothing that has not already been discovered by some person in another way. Another, more critical perspective simply understands channeling as a form of intuition to which someone wants to lend a special authority by presenting himself or herself as the source of a spiritual entity. However, the channelers understand the content of their channeling to be important messages from spiritual entities that actually exist.

As a form of establishing contact with spiritual and/or spirit beings, channeling already has a long tradition in a certain sense. For example, the Koran was transmitted to the Prophet Mohammed through the Archangel Gabriel as a message from Allah to be given to the people. In other religions as well, this phenomenon is quite well-known: For example, in Tibetan Buddhism the technique of channeling is used for various purposes such as the role of the State Oracle in Nechung for finding the respective new Dalai Lama. Shamanism also has numerous trance techniques with which an altered state of consciousness can be produced to establish a direct contact with the gods and spirits. And finally, some Christian churches engage in the so-called "speaking in tongues," a well-known, special manifestation of religious rapture that is considered the main evidence that the Holy Spirit has "descended upon the people."

Channeling can occur in very different ways for the medium. Sometimes there may be a physical change, possibly a change in the sound of the voice or it may assume a different rhythm than usual. Some mediums fall into a deep trance, others remain more or less conscious and can therefore consciously perceive the messages during the channelings. All channeling sessions are usually recorded so that the messages can be listened to again afterward and written down, if so desired.

One especially significant factor in channeled messages is that in addition to their contents, there is also an inherent "guidance of the energy" within them—meaning the way in which the individual words are organized into sentences. The "guidance of the energy" generally aims to increase the energetic vibration of the message's recipient. Seen in this way, a medium is more than just a channel but always also a type of interpreter for messages from the spiritual world. In the perception of many mediums, the spiritual entities do not even give them concrete words or sentences but images, thought impulses, and "energetic data." In turn, the medium fills these with substance and then dresses them in the words that correspond most closely with the energetic message.

One problem that sometimes arises in channeling is the undiscussable nature of the messages received. In terms of the content of their channeling, mediums usually cite higher entities beyond themselves. We can speak with a physically present spiritual teacher who makes a certain statement and possibly even express criticism. This may develop into a conversation from which both people can profit. But an individual cannot discuss a message from the spiritual world with the medium since the higher entity is usually not available for a conversation.

As in other areas of spirituality, channeling is always concerned with finding out for ourselves what is actually good for us. In this process, it is especially important to never give up our individual responsibility and, above all, never to blindly follow the advice of a spiritual entity without being in contact with our innermost self.

Speaking from the Heart

Sabine Fennell writes about her path with Reiki and her work as a channeler:
"I have been connected with Reiki since 1990 and have been a Reiki Master/Teacher since 1993. Within about four years, I initiated around 70 people and then left this traditional track in the outside world. In my Reiki Box, I once placed the desire of reaching and opening other hearts through words that are spoken from the heart. At that time, I did not yet know that I would become a channeler—mainly through purposeful meditation. This task has filled me with the greatest joy since 1996."[3]

In addition to the channeling sessions, according to Sabine Fennell, she also performs psychic consultations, trainings, and emotional-body therapy. Above all, this work involves developing the inner senses and learning to draw from one's own heart source. For her, Reiki is a "door-opener for inner abilities, creative processes, and more perception with all of the senses."[4]

When I asked Sabine whether she wanted to contribute a channeled text to this book, she was immediately open for it. I am pleased that the text on page 226, the record of a message channeled by Sabine Fennell on July 9, 2004, has become a part of this book.

⌒

Straightening Up

I had another profound experience that went beyond the boundaries of my previous experiences with Reiki in a spinal-column straightening facilitated by the spiritual healer and Reiki Master/Teacher Dieter Reimer. Through Christian Stippekohl, who organized the straightenings for Dieter Reimer in Berlin at that time, I learned about the possibility of having a scoliotic pelvis corrected within a few seconds through the power of divine interaction so that the spinal column can straighten itself again. Since I, like almost every human being, had a slightly scoliotic pelvis, I became curious.

As I knew, Dieter Reimer had been trained by the well-known healer and Reiki Master/Teacher Pjotr Elkunoviz. Shortly after the conversation with Christian Stippekohl, I saw a television report on the healing work of Pjotr Elkunoviz and his wife, Anne Hübner, who is also a healer and Reiki Master/Teacher, as well as a medium. In the report that was broadcast in the series *"Wunderheiler"* (Miracle Healers) on the ARD station[5], many people appeared on camera to confirm the effectiveness of this simple and successful form of spinal-column straightening. Even the members of the television team apparently were so convinced of the effectiveness of this form of treatment that they also had the straightenings done. A few days later, I signed up for this type of straightening, which was scheduled to take place in Berlin.

The procedure of the straightening itself seems surprisingly simple. I laid myself down on a table; Dieter Reimer raised one hand, appeared to be saying something in thought, and performed a brief movement. It felt like I was surrounded by a bell of energy, and then it was already over. When I stood up again, I immediately noticed how my posture, my entire existence in my body had fundamentally changed. On the basis of the marks on my heels that were made before the straightening, I could clearly recognize that the balancing of my scoliotic pelvis had been successful. I could hardly believe it. After the straightening, I also received a Reiki treatment that was very good for me and enveloped me in soft, flowing energy.

Divine Gift

Pjotr Elkunoviz and the healers who he has trained have already been able to help several ten-thousands of people with their divine gift. In the summer of 2004, when I spoke with Anne Hübner, I discovered that there is a waiting list of about 15,000 people who would like to be treated by Pjotr. In the words of Christian Stippekohl, who has now also received the training to become a healer and Reiki Master/Teacher from Pjotr Elkunoviz and directs a healing center in Berlin, Pjotr sees himself as a "tool in God's hand. The help provided for humanity through him is performed by the divine spirit working through him. The straightening is the core of his beneficial work for complaints of all sorts. He has the power to correct an illness-causing scoliotic pelvis within seconds and without even touching it. (...) Pjotr Elkunoviz does not see his work as a miracle but as a law of nature that is the right of every human being. The power at work is the Absolute and helps with everything."[6]

In addition to the heart of their healing work, the spinal-column straightening, Pjotr Elkunoviz and Anne Hübner also train people in Reiki. Both of them have been working as Reiki Teachers since about 1991. Pjotr received his initiation into the Master Degree from Horst and Edith Günther. Anne was initiated into the Master Degree by Norbert and Karin Kuhl. Even before his initiation into the First Reiki Degree, Pjotr already had the ability to perform the straightenings.[7]

A part of the healing work by Pjotr and Anne is also the channelings done by Anne. In addition, Sai Baba, the well-known Indian wisdom teacher and healer, is especially significant for the healing work of the two. It is said that Sai Baba has materialized in the healing center of Anne and Pjotr on several occasions. Moreover, according to Anne Hübner, she was trained by Sai Baba in a medial way.[8]

My Path with Reiki

My personal path with Reiki has been closely connected with my interest in the Buddhist teachings from the very beginning. When I began to be interested in Reiki, my attraction to Tibetan Buddhism also awakened. Even before my initiation into the First Reiki Degree, I took refuge in Buddhism with Lama Ole Nydahl, a Tibetan-Buddhist teacher of Danish origin who has been traveling around the globe for decades and has founded many spiritual centers around the world. For some years, I visited Ole's lectures whenever he was in Berlin and loved going to the front afterward, waiting in line with the others to receive his blessing. I also attended several events with the Dalai Lama, as well as lectures and seminars by the well-known Tibetan-Buddhist teacher Sogyal Rinpoche.

About two years after I was initiated into the First Reiki Degree, there was a moment when I asked myself the question: Reiki or Buddhism? At the time, I experienced this question as an either-or decision. I wanted to commit myself to a "main spiritual teaching" for a certain amount of time since I tended to change from one thing to the next and had recognized that this did not promote my spiritual development at that point in time. Consequently, the question that I asked myself was: Should I take Paul Mitchell, with whom I could have possibly taken the training to become a Reiki Master, as a teacher or should I take the path of Tibetan Buddhism with Lama Ole Nydahl? I decided upon Paul at that time, and therefore essentially for Reiki. However, today I no longer see this as a matter of either-or. I practice and teach the Usui System of Reiki and am simultaneously close to Buddhism, practice Buddhist meditations, and maintain personal contacts to Buddhist teachers.

In the course of the years, I have become increasingly familiar with the basic characteristics of the Buddhist Teachings. The following text presents a brief overview of the essential aspects of Buddhism[9]:

What is Buddhism?

Buddhism is one of the six major world religions, along with Christianity, Islam, Hinduism, Taoism, and Confucianism. There are about 380 million Buddhists throughout the world. Buddhism understands itself as a religion without an ultimate God. Accordingly, it is not a philosophy, as people sometimes claim. It does not intend to explain the world but instead is a teaching of liberation that shows very concrete paths leading from suffering and imperfection to harmony and happiness.

At the heart of the Buddhist world view are the "Four Noble Truths": 1. Human suffering, 2. Its causes, 3. The opportunities for overcoming suffering, as well as 4. The practical means to accomplish this. The characteristics and exercises of Buddhism are ethical conduct, compassion, meditation, and deep insight. Buddhism is distinguished by tolerance, a willingness to engage in dialog, freedom from dogmas, and non-violence.

One author has written that Buddhism is "a system of practical exercises, an aligned lifestyle, and insights that can be applied at any time by any person and without dependence. It does not require any faith—just the courage to try something and examine the results yourself."[10]

A significant Buddhist scripture advises the following:

"Do not let yourself be guided by reports, by tradition, or by hearsay. Do not let yourself be guided by the authority of religious texts, nor by pure logic or conclusions, nor by paying attention to outward appearances, nor by enthusiasm for speculative opinions, nor by apparent opportunities, nor by the imagination: This is your teacher. But when you know for yourself that certain things are unhealthy, wrong, and bad, then give them up. And when you know for yourself that certain things are healthy and good, then accept them and follow them. (Vimamsaka Sutta)"[11]

The founder of this religion, Siddharta Gautama, probably also attained enlightenment in a similar way. From then on, he was called "the Buddha" by his students; this word comes from the Sanskrit language and means "the Awakened One" or "the Enlightened One." Siddharta Gautama lived about 500 years before Christ. In the course of a long spiritual search, he discovered the so-called "Path of the Middle" that lies between asceticism and sensual pleasure, balancing all extremes.

One portion of the Buddhist perspective is the teachings of reincarnation. Karma connects the existence of human beings with their previous lives. A person's karma includes both the good and the bad deeds. It is created through the chain of cause and effect. The ultimate goal of human existence is *Nirvana,* a state of inner happiness in which there is no more desire and no more karma.

As in all other religions, Buddhism also has various forms and schools. The oldest and most original form of Buddhism is Theravada Buddhism; this direction is strongly characterized by monasticism. Mahayana Buddhism developed later and is also directed toward the so-called laypeople, those who are not monks or nuns. Special forms of Buddhism are Zen Buddhism, which developed in China and fully blossomed in Japan, as well as Tibetan Buddhism.

One of the main elements of the Buddhist teaching is "the Eight-Fold Path." This includes right insight, right decision, right speech, right action, right way of life, right striving, right awareness, and right contemplation. Further aspects of these eight fundamental types of conduct are recorded in great detail in extensive scriptures.

There are five basic vows for practitioners of Buddhism. These are:

"I vow to abstain from killing,
I vow to abstain from stealing,
I vow to abstain from the incorrect way of life that indulges in sensual pleasure,
I vow to abstain from lying,
I vow to abstain from intoxication.

Abstaining from evil,
Commitment to do good actions,
Cleansing one's own senses,
This is what the Buddha teaches.
(Dhammapada 183)"[12]

New Contact

Some years after my initiation into the Master Degree, I met with Swami Prem Jagran for the first time. He came to Berlin in regular intervals, where he taught *Ngal So Chag Wang Reiki,* a Buddhist form of Reiki. My motivation for the meeting was to discover more about "Buddhist Reiki" and perhaps do an interview with him for the *Reiki Magazin.* However, at our first meeting I received very little concrete information. But the days following the meeting were quite wonderful for me. I felt how this somehow had to be related to the strong, healing charisma of Swami Prem Jagran.

When he returned to the city some weeks later, we had another meeting. In the meantime, I began to also become personally interested in *Ngal So Chag Wang Reiki.* Jagran offered me the possibility of being part of a First Degree seminar as a guest. I took advantage of this opportunity a few weeks later. The hoped-for interview for the *Reiki Magazin* also took place in the fall of 2003 and was generally well-received upon publication.

Buddhist Roots?

A question that concerns many Reiki practitioners is if the Usui System of Reiki basically has Buddhist origins. Hawayo Takata had pointed out a correlation between the Usui System and Buddhist scriptures on a number of occasions.[13]

Furthermore, the Reiki Master Ray Pine reported in an article published in the *Reiki Magazine International* on his visit to Borobudur, the largest area with historical Buddhist structures in the world, located in Indonesia. He saw ancient, symbolic depictions carved in stone here, which are strongly reminiscent of people practicing Reiki. He writes the following about them:

"The main part of the pictograph shows a person who is either ill or has led such a good life that he is being rewarded. This person is surrounded by other people putting their hands on him (or her). A person at the back is clearly putting both hands on the receiver's head; other hands can be seen on the shoulders, and there are hands on the person's body and legs. It looks like a Buddhist group Reiki treatment!"[14]

Walter Lübeck also sees a correlation between the roots of the Usui System and Buddhist scriptures:

"Dr. Usui belonged to various spiritual groups and researched many different techniques of healing with the life energy through laying on hands. The idea that the divine healing power is transmitted directly through the body of the healer, through the hands to those who need healing, impressed him very much. In this process, it was always very important for the healer to prepare accordingly using exercises to keep the energy channels clean and collect an adequate supply of *Ki* so that the healings do not use the body's reserves, which are vital for life. This was naturally very time-consuming and rather unsuitable for laypeople. At the beginning of the 1920s, probably in the texts of esoteric Buddhism, he found that the monk Kukai had brought techniques corresponding with these methods more than a thousand years earlier from China to Japan."[15]

In addition to Hawayo Takata, Ray Pine, and Walter Lübeck, a correlation between the roots of the Usui System and Buddhist scriptures has also been seen by Don Alexander (cf. pg. 33), Dr. Ranga Premaratna (cf. pg. 124), and many other Reiki Masters/ Teachers.

When I asked Swami Prem Jagran within the scope of the interview for the *Reiki Magazin* whether he knows if there are Buddhist scriptures that show a correlation between the Usui System of Reiki and Buddhist Reiki systems, he cited the scriptures of the Medicine Buddha in the "Higher Tantra Yoga of Naropa, in the Tantra of the Secret Initiations."[16]

Ngal So Chag Wang Reiki

Ngal So Chag Wang Reiki is a Tibetan-Buddhist system of Reiki. Tibetan Buddhism is a Tantric teaching. Tantra is a word from the Sanskrit language and means "weave, thread, chain."[17] A direct translation of the word "Tantra" is also "energetic, mental continuum"[18]. As we see, the original meaning of the word has little relation to how it is used today in the West (as a general term for the techniques of ritual sexual unification more or less based on Tantricism).

Tantricism is a religious teaching in Hinduism and Buddhism that developed in the First Century A.D., aimed at establishing the contact with the divine through rituals and ceremonies. For this purpose, it uses magical means such as mantras (see pg. 220), *yantras* (meditation diagrams and drawings), *bijas* (Sanskrit: seeds; the energies that are inherent in every material manifestation) and *mudras* (Sanskrit: seal, mystery; symbolic gestures of the fingers or hands).[19] A main characteristic of Tantric practice is that the energy of suffering and aggression is directly transformed into spiritual awakening.[20]

Ngal So Chag Wang Reiki was brought to life by the great Tibetan-Buddhist teacher and healer T.Y.S. Lama Gangchen Tulku Rinpoche. According to Swami Prem Jagran, Lama Gangchen has been in a pure transmission lineage for many lifetimes in the tradition of the Gelugpa, one of the four main lineages of Tibetan Buddhism.[21] The spiritual lineage of *Ngal So Chag Wang Reiki* goes directly back to the Buddha. When I asked Swami Prem Jagran for the literal translation of *Ngal So Chag Wang Reiki,* he responded as follows:

"Ngal is related to everything that can become dirty, no matter what it is, both the outside and the inside. *So* is the solution for this state of contamination. This not only means cleansing what has already been soiled but also preventing the soiling. *Chag Wang* means 'the hand of the Buddha.' *Chag* is the hand, and *Wang* represents the Buddha. And when you ask what does Reiki mean, you must admit that you do not know. So how can we interpret *Ngal So Chag Wang Reiki?* It should allow us to become aware that we are now causing harm in both the internal and the external. If we become truly conscious of this, and we are seriously concerned with it, then we should not let our consciousness continually be focused on this problem but instead find a solution through the *So. Chag Wang* is the hand of the Buddha. When we turn to the Buddha, then our thoughts are always focused on Shakyamuni, meaning to this enlightened person. Yet, I am certain that each of us has the potential to become a Buddha. But we must work at it.

We must be responsible in order to achieve this. Each of us can use the hand of the Buddha by uniting our own energies with those of the universe in order to find a solution, the *So*, for the problem of the contamination, meaning the *Ngal*. As in the Orient, *Ngal So Chag Wang* is actually read from right to left."[22]

Moreover, Swami Prem Jagran explains:

"Lama Gangchen said that *Ngal So Chag Wang Reiki* knows eight levels or degrees; however, these are not eight technical levels but eight levels of consciousness. (...) Of these eight levels or degrees, there are five in which the initiations are performed between the Lama and me, and three take place through self-initiation. There are, for example, 22 ways of giving the mental treatment."[23]

Swami Prem Jagran teaches the first levels of *Ngal So Chag Wang Reiki* in the familiar structure of the three degrees according to the Usui System of Reiki: First Degree, Second Degree, and Master Degree. After these, additional levels of *Ngal So Chag Wang Reiki* are taught in the respectively appropriate structures.[24]

The Life Path of a Healer

Already in his childhood, Swami Prem Jagran had the gift of helping others by laying his hands on them: "Since just over the age of six years, I have been laying my hands directly on the sick parts of both people and animals. This perception of 'seeing and feeling' is natural for me, in so far as I never had to learn to do it as it was something I was born able to do. Throughout my whole life I have been in continuous contact with a part of me from which I have been able to draw knowledge and wisdom. In the first ten years of my life in particular, I had visions and received audible instructions (which I later realised to be particular 'symbols' or 'signs') to use for the various sicknesses which I would meet during my journey as a healer."[25]

The Energy of Breath

Taoist Exercise as directed by Swami Prem Jagran

I advise you to carry out this simple but effective exercise before you practice Reiki or other forms of energetic meditation.

Kneel down in Seiza, the Japanese posture, keeping the back straight. Keep the shoulders relaxed and the hands resting on the thighs with the palms of the hands facing upwards.

Close your eyes and draw your attention to your breathing.

After a few (3 or 4) long, deep breaths, using the belly more than the shoulders while inhaling, close the palms of the hands over the thumbs.

During this action you should breathe in air through your nose.

Holding your breath and keeping the hands closed, contract the muscles of the buttocks to close the anus.
This contraction will help you to raise the back.

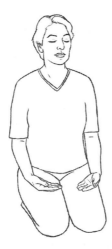

Sitting Relaxed

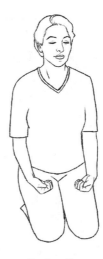

Contracting

Continue this movement and you will find yourself in a kneeling position.

As the body rises, the hands move away from the body and open suddenly towards the sky above your head and at the same time the inhaled air is expelled.

The air is expelled from the mouth, pronouncing the sound of the letter A (AH).

The complete cycle of the exercise as described above should be repeated 7 (seven) times and no more.

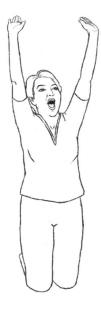

Opening

In the Spring of 2000, Swami Prem Jagran met for the first time with Lama Gangchen Tulku Rinpoche. Shortly thereafter, according to Swami Prem Jagran, "on the 7th July 2000 (the day of his birthday) Lama Gangchen announced that he wanted to give a gift to the population of this planet: He said 'I want to give you the complete method of Reiki!' (...) And so it came about that he gave life to a new, pure lineage which he called *Ngal So Chag Wang Reiki*, and I, together with other friends, received the direct initiation."[26]

"One of the most significant points of this method," Swami Prem Jagran writes, "which struck me, was the possibility to use ancient systems of tantric purification, which have been simplified for us Westerners and which permit our inner environment, the relationship with the elements and the chakras, to return to their completely pure status which is then in an ideal state to receive the energy of the pure lineage."[27]

"For me," according to Swami Prem Jagran, *"Ngal So Chag Wang Reiki* has been a form of 'illuminating meditation' and it has an incredible strength of inner acceleration."[28] After he had previously practiced the Usui System of Reiki for many years, he came to the conclusion: "As it is, practising Reiki is something extraordinary. It is the beginning of a very beautiful inner journey ... but personally, after having experimented with *Ngal So Chag Wang Reiki,* I believe that Usui's method was missing 'something'."[29]

In a previously unpublished interview that I had with Swami Prem Jagran, he said the following about giving Reiki and the differences he feels there are between the Usui System of Reiki and *Ngal So Chag Wang Reiki:*

"When I give Reiki, I do not have a goal. I simply let it happen. I try to let Reiki flow. In the process, I often come into a state where I remember something that we have forgotten. It is the feeling of having a home. It is the moment when something happens, the calm and the peace. At the beginning of my Reiki practice, I obviously had other sensations. At the start, I concentrated more on how Reiki feels, how warm it is or how cold. Or I saw images. But now that I have met Lama Gangchen and *Ngal So Chag Wang Reiki,* I can feel the 'fragrance of emptiness'."[30]

The Essence of Healing

After the encounter with Lama Gangchen Tulku Rinpoche, Swami Prem Jagran took refuge in Buddhism and received many blessings and basic Tibetan-Buddhist initiations in the following period of time, especially from Lama Gangchen and also from the Dalai Lama. In February of 2000, the royal family in Nepal officially recognized him as a spiritual healer after he had successfully treated the queen mother.[31]

I was present as an interpreter at some of the healing consultations that Swami Prem Jagran gave in Berlin, which offered me the opportunity of experiencing his healing work close up. As a result, I discovered that in addition to the very special abilities that a spiritual healer must obviously possess, the essence of healing work is basically very simple. In my experience, above all this basically involves personal attention, openness, and a certain simplicity in dealing with people who are seeking help; furthermore, it means truly seeing them with their problems, accepting them, and ultimately using this basis in a healing way, depending on the methods or abilities, to influence them with the actual goal of awakening their own powers of self-healing.

Holistic Nature

I very much value my personal contact with Jagran and am pleased that he wants to open a healing center in Berlin. One of his main concerns is working together with physicians and scientists toward following a holistic approach in healing work. In cooperation with the traditional sciences, he would like to prove that human beings do not just consist of their bodies but also require complementary support on the spiritual level in addition to the usual medical care in order to complete the process of becoming healthy and healing.

The practical exercise on page 242 was given to me by Swami Prem Jagran for this book. According to Jagran, this is "one of the five secret exercises of Taoist monks" that he has put into his own words here.

Crossing Paths

Another person who I have encountered on my path with Reiki and with whom I feel very connected is Peter Mascher. I met Peter for the first time at a Reiki event with Phyllis Furumoto and Paul Mitchell in Cologne. About a year later, we met again in Berlin and used the time for an extensive exchange of ideas. A short time later, Peter became a student of Phyllis Furumoto in order to take the Master training with her. We met again at the first "H'Art& Soul" Festival that took place in 2001 in the Lüneburg Heath, Germany. Peter is a professional instrumentalist (he plays viola in a Dutch orchestra), and he headed a workshop on musical improvisation at the festival.

About one year later, we met again at a seminar with Don Alexander in Chemnitz, Germany. Peter had begun to intensively examine the history of the Usui System. I noticed how much he felt drawn to Don Alexander as a teacher at the same time that he was a Master Candidate with Phyllis Furumoto. We talked for an entire night about his dilemma, and I supported him in making a decision. When we talked on the phone some time later, Peter said that he had now begun the Master training with Don. He told me how much he valued Don's heart-felt attention and the meditative practice of his teaching, and that he felt a great love for him that he could not put into words.

We now have extensive phone conversations with each other at longer intervals of time to talk about Reiki and life in general. In the meantime, Peter has told me that he has become familiar with the Process Work according to Arnold Mindell, about which he is very enthusiastic. This form of the work, according to Peter, has its roots in the dream work developed by C. G. Jung.

In the spring of 2004, Peter received the initiation into the Master Degree from Don Alexander. Shortly thereafter, he traveled to Japan with Don for three weeks. We finally met in the summer of 2004 in St. Peter Ording to once again spend some time together. The two of us have a very interesting connection: On the one hand, the paths that we have taken appear to be very different; yet, these paths seem to be constantly crossing again since new points of contact keep developing. This is a very remarkable dynamic!

I am happy that Peter has contributed the exercise on the topic of "Reiki and Process Work" on the following pages to this book.

Process Oriented Movement Meditation
By Peter Mascher

I am now sitting on my cushion and begin with Hatsureiho, a light meditation, but my mind and body just do not want to become still. I am in turmoil. When I try to calmly let everything pass by me, I start to boil inside. I feel tension in my muscles, and a film runs in front of my inner eye. I want to jump up and scream.

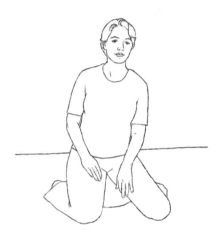

Perceiving the Reluctance

I stop this film right here for a moment and look at myself from all sides.
We usually express ourselves in "channels," which we often just perceive subconsciously. For example, channels are feelings, body movements, inner images and sounds, voices, and even inner figures that want to make contact with us. All of these are part of our dreaming body, which we live with 24 hours a day, whether we perceive it or not. Sometimes what we perceive within us is very fine and concealed; but at other times everything within us screams and we become afraid of ourselves.
My experience is that even after years of meditation practice, it is precisely this "dream body" that would like to play with me time and again. It simply does not leave my thoughts alone—it appears to be a part of my soul.

What we usually call "thoughts" is in reality a complex process of arising inner images and figures with which we also constantly have dialogs on the physical level. It is often difficult to just let go of all of these impulses in a meditation. If we do not succeed at this, we can also take other paths and "ride our horse backwards."

A process oriented meditation begins with the greatest respect for ourselves and with gratitude for everything that is. Within this context, the word "process" is not used here for the types of behaviors and problems with which we are quite familiar within us and can also name. Instead, this means looking at the processes of the moment, whatever would like to take form, even if the impulse for it is still very small. I allow myself to dream while I am awake.

Let's start the exercise:

Your best teacher is your own perception. So allow yourself now to perceive your dreaming body. Do not control yourself. Let everything live as it feels at the moment. If you feel pain in your body, then go exactly to where it is and let yourself be moved by what is. Feel your way into the pain or the tension. Where is it in your body? You may want to leave your meditation posture and move as your body desires in this moment. Do not be afraid to make sounds, and also perceive the fine impulses, the points where you do not feel well.

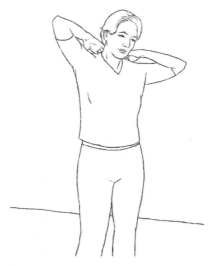

Feeling the Way into the Tension

If you do not feel any movement at all within you, then look within yourself to see whether there are images within you that would like to be lived. Sometimes this is just a feeling and the image comes later. Trust in yourself and give yourself time. Feel whether these images can be set into motion and which figures arise in the process. In case everything clearly points in this direction, have the courage to play these figures. If your perception is still very cautious, then permit yourself to enlarge all of the small impulses. Be thankful and open yourself for everything that IS. If nothing happens in the movement channel, then simply refocus your attention and search for an image or a feeling. Always begin wherever your attention leads you on its own. Everything that IS at the moment is good and valuable and leads you into your dream figure. Perceive them and play them in your dream theater until you can better understand and accept them. Perceive how the pain and tensions, movements, and inner images change in an almost playful way. Like a child, be astonished at yourself.

You may also encounter figures on your dream journey that are unpleasant for you. These are often people who have hurt you at some point and who you now encounter again within yourself. Have the courage to listen to them and not run away. It may be that your body is hurting in silence because you would like to run away from them and from yourself.

A few explanations about this:

In this work, there are no givens from the outside. I am my own best teacher and therefore retain the entire authority in my process. Listening to the smallest impulse and enlarging it means "amplification." Sometimes following the inner images and then expressing the same thing in the voice or in movement means following a "change of channel." When we do this, we experience a daydream, a dream figure that speaks within us. We can only find inner peace when we have listened to ourselves and allowed our "dream body" to live within us.

Returning to the exercise:

You suddenly feel that you have no more desire to continue. The energy fades and a resistance arises within you. You have reached the limit in the exercise. This limit must be respected and perceived in a precise way. Who is standing on this boundary and does not permit you to go any further? Can you translate your feelings into images and movement, looking somewhat beyond this boundary? Everyone feels ridiculous at some point when we do things that are apparently beyond our possibilities or appear unacceptable to us, or when we perceive this for the first time. With complete love for yourself, permit yourself to look somewhat behind this boundary. Who is blocking you there in your dream world? Have the courage to even look into unpleasant feelings, and then return to the movement. The energy behind this could be very valuable for you. Can you accept and become more familiar with this "boundary figure" and its energies? Have the courage to play with it and pay special attention while you do this to your fine perception of small impulses, whether these are movement, images, feelings, or language and sound.

Is this person perhaps a part of yourself that is completely new to you? Respect everything that you feel and experience, and trust in your own intuition during your inner journey. Do not exceed your limits, and stop the exercise when you do not feel any more energy for continuing with it. Allow yourself a moment of quiet and perceive how the energy is moving within you. If you like, make a drawing of one of the dream figures within you that arises time and again. Then give it a name. Figures will not always arise. If this is the case, then simply name your momentary feeling and make a little drawing of it, if that helps you. Value everything that is there right now.

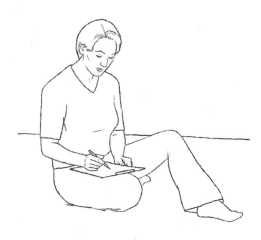

Making a Drawing

If you have worked while standing or walking, sit back down again and enjoy the peace arising within you. Allow yourself an inner smile, and now begin with a light meditation such as Hatsureiho, if you like. Let yourself fall into the Reiki energy as you do this.

Summary:

When we permit ourselves to dream with our entire body, with all the feelings, images, and movements, then we experience our "dream body." It is a part of our personality and our soul that we ordinarily hardly perceive in everyday life. When we seek stillness, it suddenly draws attention to itself and sometimes even screams inwardly. When we learn to accept it and live it, Reiki will begin to flow more freely within and we slowly come to peace. Then we no longer have shadow battles with ourselves, and our mindfulness and gratitude toward ourselves and everything that lives within us will grow.

It requires courage to intensify the things that disturb us or are unpleasant for us. And yet, this is the key to success. Always just go as far as you would like to. All of the possibilities cited here are just examples of a work in which your own creativity and the respect for yourself decides everything on its own. Your love for yourself is the essence on the path to your very personal, inner peace.

9. Spirituality
The Search for Something Higher

In the description of the Usui System of Reiki according to Phyllis Furumoto, it essentially has four aspects: It is a healing method, it promotes personal development, it is (and requires) spiritual discipline, and it creates a mystic order.[1]

As I already mentioned above, my approach to the Usui System of Reiki came through spirituality. Even before my initiation into the First Reiki Degree, I had been involved with spirituality and esotericism for many years. However, this was more on the mental level with the help of systems such as Tarot and astrology. Through Reiki, it became possible for me to directly experience spirituality. It inspired me, and now I have already been giving myself Reiki on a regular basis for more than ten years in order to lastingly maintain the connection with the universal life energy and continuously intensify it.

In the course of the years, as I began to increasingly question my concepts of the world and life, I also became more interested in the question as to what is the essence of spirituality. One day, I found the following enlightening excerpt in an esoteric dictionary:

"Spirituality is understood as going beyond or questioning the obvious or sensory material world. This presumes that there is a pure consciousness beyond the individual consciousness of human beings and/or that there must be a spiritual world beyond the material. This crossing of the boundaries is also interpreted as the liberation and self-realization of a human being. Spirituality itself is the object of esoteric teachings and systems and all religions."[2]

This brief and succinct definition summarizes the fundamental aspects of spirituality:

1. Going beyond and/or questioning the material world—the fundamental core of spiritual activity.

2. The existence of a pure consciousness and/or a spiritual world beyond the material world—the starting point for spiritual thought.

3. The liberation and/or self-realization that can be achieved when we have a spiritual orientation in life.

Furthermore, the definition points out the greater context within which spirituality is significant. Spirituality is shown to be the heart of all esoteric teachings and systems, as well as every religion; in a certain sense, this makes it the very basis of all esotericism and all religions. The Bible, the Koran, the Talmud, the Bhagavad-Gita, and the teachings of Buddha are basically all about one thing: imparting spirituality. And not just there, but also in astrology, anthroposophy, energy work, all of the esoteric disciplines are ultimately concerned with conveying spirituality, which means a spiritual way of thinking, spiritual experiences, and a spiritual lifestyle.

⌐

During the past 20 years, millions of people throughout the world have found access to a spiritual way of life through the Usui System of Reiki or have spiritual experiences with Reiki that touched them deeply. Seen in this light, the Usui System of Reiki can be called a spiritual system.

If the Usui System of Reiki is spiritual in its nature, we can ask the question: Does it tend to have the characteristics of an esoteric teaching or does it actually have aspects of a religious community? The following pages are dedicated to this question, which various scholars of religious studies are also exploring. The first section will look at the nature of esoteric teachings and compare them with the Usui System, followed by a brief description of the distinguishing features of a religion and how they also compare with the Usui System.

What is Esotericism?

"Esotericism" describes an area that has neither a clear contour nor one standard definition. This has resulted in the colloquial use of the term esotericism expanding its meaning to describe every possible area including natural methods of healing, various forms of therapy, and Far Eastern martial arts. In order to get a closer picture of this word, it may be helpful to not understand esotericism as a term that outlines or even tries to define an area but see it instead as a designation for a certain way of thinking. This way of thinking reveals increasingly more of its true nature the more we become involved with disciplines that have an esoteric orientation.

According to the Greek root, esotericism means: "directly inward" or "turned within." So we can probably say that esoteric teachings and systems are essentially concerned with looking inward. They have the goal of recognizing one's own nature and self-realization.

The knowledge and the practices that are used for this purpose are also directed inward in the sense that they are not intended for "the whole world" but are respectively just accessible to a certain group of people. In view of this fact and the variety of esoteric disciplines, the following question naturally arises: What is the common denominator of all these different teachings and systems that are accessible respectively only to a certain group of people? What defines them as esoteric teachings or systems?

Here is the attempt at a definition on the basis of many books on the topic:

Esoteric teachings and systems generally include the following aspects, among others:

- The preservation of a specific spiritual tradition that dates back to a founder or founder community.

- Teachings—meaning commentaries—by the teacher or master that are directed to the students and/or course participants.

- Initiations within the scope of the step-by-step progression within the system and/or the teachings.

- The use of symbols—within the scope of the respective practices—or generally symbolic acts in correlation with the system and/or the teachings.

- A certain degree of secrecy in relation to the knowledge or the practices that form the heart of the system and/or the teachings.

Today, the last aspect is somewhat weakened by the fact that a large portion of knowledge that was previously kept secret is now basically available to anyone through its publication in the modern media. However, this knowledge is ultimately worthless without the corresponding explanations and/or initiations from an authorized teacher so these types of publications do not harm the principle of secrecy that is inherent in the esoteric way of thinking.

The fact is, as is aptly described in a book on the topic of esotericism, that no access to a symbol, a mythos, or a world of reality can be gained without personal effort toward a step-by-step, progressive explanation.[3]

In other words: In relation to esoteric knowledge, this does not involve the simple acquisition of knowledge in the same sense as applies to the school or university; instead, it involves continuous personal effort and contact with a teacher we trust in order to discover progressive access to a new world of reality—a world that lies beyond our given, material world. And such an access is not at all possible without the relationship to a teacher, without whose step-by-step explanations and initiations that he or she performs in accordance with the respective tradition—and, above all, without the personal efforts on the part of the person who is willing to learn about all these things.[4]

The Usui System as an Esoteric Discipline?

When considering this overview of the distinguishing features of esoteric teachings: Can we now say that the Usui System of Reiki is an esoteric discipline? To answer this question, it appears helpful to once more examine the main characteristics and see how they resonate with the Usui System of Reiki:

- *The preservation of a specific spiritual tradition that dates back to a founder or a founder community.*

This characteristic can be affirmed in principle for the Usui System of Reiki. However, as described in Chapter 1 (pg. 35), in the Usui

System of Reiki we have the unusual situation that the founder of the system hardly had a lasting, form-giving influence on the system that he established—at least in terms of the current expressions of the system with its immensely varied forms—in contrast to comparable esoteric disciplines. However, the various forms and styles of the Usui System that we encounter today basically have the same elements and they all derive their spiritual lineage from Mikao Usui. Seen from this perspective, this characteristic can basically be affirmed for the Usui System of Reiki. Yet, we should give consideration to whether it would be more appropriate to see Mikao Usui as the person who established it rather than as the founder (cf. pg. 36/265).

- *Teachings—meaning commentaries—by the teacher or master that are directed to the students and/or course participants.*

This aspect is a component of the Usui System of Reiki. In Reiki seminars and at Reiki-exchange meetings, the Master/Teacher answers questions from the students and explains the correlations within the system.

- *Initiations within the scope of the step-by-step progression within the system.*

This is also a component of the Usui System of Reiki. When learning each of the degrees or each level, one (or more) initiation(s) are performed respectively. This applies comprehensively to all of the forms and styles of the system.

- *The use of symbols or generally symbolic acts in correlation with the system.*

These two aspects are also components of the Usui System of Reiki. Beginning with the Second Degree, practitioners use symbols for purposes such as mental treatment or distant treatment with Reiki. Masters/Teachers use symbols in the initiation rituals. The use of symbols applies to all of the forms and styles of the systems. In terms of the aspect of "general symbolic acts," this may be more or less pronounced depending upon the tradition and/or the Master/ Teacher. As can be observed, this aspect of their actions frequently remains unconscious for many Masters/Teachers, even if it is quite pronounced.

- *A certain degree of secrecy in relation to the knowledge or the practices that form the heart of the system.*

This aspect is a component of the Usui System of Reiki as well. The knowledge about the symbols and practices of the respective higher degrees is usually subject to a certain extent of secrecy. Even after the publication of the symbols of the Second Degree and the Master Degree in some books, it is still obvious that the greater majority of the Masters/Teachers still keep a considerable amount of their knowledge secret in terms of the advanced degrees and developmental levels around those who have not been initiated into these degrees or have not (yet) reached these levels of development. This applies to almost every form and style of the system, whereby the degree of secrecy is more or less pronounced depending on the school.

Summary: The main characteristics of esoteric disciplines apply largely to the Usui System of Reiki. Seen in this way, the Usui System can be called a system with esoteric attributes.

What is Religion?

The origin of the word "religion" is unclear. There are various Latin words that could be the basis of this term. Theses are:

- *religari* = reconnecting with God or the connection of the visible with the invisible world in which mysterious forces work whose favor must be attained.

- *relegere* = the conscientious respect for what is a part of worshipping the divine.

- *religio* = religious awe, piety

In its nature, religion is a response of human beings to their life situation. In the confrontation with the problems of this world, people attempt to develop an understanding of the universe and its existence in order to give their lives significance and a goal. Religion, according to one expert in this field, has the effect of explaining, confirming the status quo and legitimizing the social order. It creates security in the conflicts with the world and promotes the solidarity of the religious community.[5]

A central element of every religion is priesthood. The priest, in simplified terms, is the mediator between the believers or the religious community and the divine. He is the authorized representative of the religious community in such activities as prayer and sacrifice and is considered the keeper of the knowledge. During the course of development of religions, we can observe that the priesthood grows into an increasingly powerful group that is increasingly dedicated to organization of the respective religion. By the same token, the priesthood has a powerful position within the societies that feel close to the respective religion.

Even if is ultimately no conclusive definition of religion because of the complexity of the associated correlations, I would like to risk a definition here—on the basis of numerous books written on this subject:

Religions generally include the following aspects, among others:

- A teaching, a belief system, a philosophy that offers a comprehensive explanation of reality; this is accompanied by the belief in supernatural beings and/or forces.

- Ethics, which means specific concepts of values and norms of behavior.

- Certain rules and regulations, such as dress and food regulations.

- Rituals such as worship services, initiations, celebrations, and prayers; the use of symbols is part of the rituals; among other things, the rituals serve the experience of transcendence.

- Myths, meaning stories about God and/or the gods, creation, and salvation, the circumstances of how the respective religion developed, and others.

- Sacred scriptures in which the respective teachings, philosophy, ethics, rules, regulations, rituals, and myths, among other things, are recorded.

- A founding figure such as Buddha in Buddhism.

- An institution, meaning an organization that has been created for practicing the respective religion.

- Sacred places, meaning cult places and/or buildings, as well as holy days such as the Advent period in Christianity.

In the life of every human being, according to a fundamental thought of the religious view of the world, there are moments when we require the accompaniment of religious rituals. These are essentially a person's birth (which is connected with naming the individual), puberty (which brings religious coming of age with it), possibly marriage (which represents a new form of connection in life), and ultimately death (which is accompanied by the person's funeral).

Over time, the fundamental differences between many religions have given rise to a problem of human coexistence. It can frequently be observed, probably because of the life-encompassing orientation that is inherent to a religion, that a religious community considers its own belief to be the only true one or sees it as the highest form of expressing the absolute truth. This may occur because every religious community considers the respective viewpoints and practices to have a certain claim to absoluteness. If this claim is projected through the community into the surrounding world, to other people, problems can arise in how its members coexist with others.

In such a case, it may help to keep in mind that the highest truth can never lie within viewpoints or contents developed by human beings but is ultimately to be found in a completely different place. One expert sees the situation like this: "The great pious ones of all religions who have thought about the relationship of the religions with each other and their relationship with the truth have not expressed their knowledge in abstract terms but in images and parables."[6]

Such an image expressing a perception of the nature of religion and the various religions with each other is the following, which comes from a poem of Zen Buddhism:

> "One and the same moon reflects
> In all waters
> All of the moons in the water
> Are one in the one single moon."[7]

The Usui System as a Religion?

To answer the question about the extent to which the Usui System of Reiki exhibits the traits of a religious community, it appears helpful to once again look at the main characteristics of religion and examine how they are reflected in the Usui System of Reiki:

- *A teaching, a belief system, a philosophy that offers a comprehensive explanation of reality; this is accompanied by the belief in supernatural beings and/or forces.*
The Usui System of Reiki is not comprised of type of generic teachings, belief system, or world view. We only observe a distinctive philosophy or view of the world in some of the forms of the system that have experienced further development. However, the belief in supernatural powers as a characteristic of how practitioners of the Usui System think can be basically affirmed; this applies, above all, in relation to the fact that the central procedure of initiation in the Usui System can hardly be explained in any other way than with the existence of supernatural powers.

- *Ethics, which means specific concepts of values and norms of behavior.*
With the Reiki Principles, the Usui System of Reiki has its own little system of rules of behavior intended to serve spiritual development. The goal of the Reiki Principles is to lead serious practitioners to their themes and contents for the purpose of both reflection and concrete translation into action. However, the principles are not intended as rules that must absolutely be observed but more as guidelines for personal spiritual development. The Reiki Principles are, in their various respective forms, a component of all of the traditions and directions of the Usui System.

- *Certain rules and regulations, such as dress and food regulations.*
There are no regulations in terms of dress or specific foods within the Usui System of Reiki. A Master/Teacher may advise his or her students to abstain from alcohol or meat on the days of the initiations or in the period directly before or after. Some individuals also express the opinion that the teacher and students should wear light-colored clothing at the initiations. However, these are just individual cases; there are no predominant teachings regarding these points.

In terms of the Reiki Principles, these should be understood as guidelines for continued spiritual development instead of rules.

- *Rituals such as worship services, initiations, celebrations, and prayers; the use of symbols is part of the rituals; among other things, the rituals serve the experience of transcendence.*
There are various rituals that are a component of the Usui System of Reiki. A very essential ritual for the form of the system is the initiation, sometimes also called attunement; at its heart, this is a form of initiation. At least one of these initiation rituals is performed in connection with every degree of the system. In addition, there is a "culture of coming together" in the Usui System of Reiki. Forms of the practitioners' frequent wish to have mutual experiences are the many Reiki-exchange meetings organized by the Masters/Teachers in which a group Reiki treatment usually takes place. In addition, there are many regional and national meetings of practitioners and Masters/Teachers with each other that may also be open to various directions. Within the scope of the initiation rituals, the Masters/Teachers use symbols. This applies to the large majority of all forms and styles of the system. The initiation ritual, as well as the group treatments, serve the experience of transcendence, among other things.

- *Myths, meaning stories about God and/or the gods, creation, and salvation, the circumstances of how the respective religion developed, and others.*

We could say that the Usui System of Reiki has a central myth. This consists of the legendary story of the system (cf. pg. 9). This story transports few facts but is traditionally told in a legendary manner by the Masters/Teachers. However, the legendary telling of the story is not a component of all forms of the Usui System. In the course of discovering new information about the beginning period of the Usui System, some Masters/Teachers are currently dispensing with telling the legendary form of the story, generally because they had long considered the information that it contains to be fact and are now disappointed that this apparently does not apply to some of it.

- *Sacred scriptures in which the respective teachings, philosophy, ethics, rules, regulations, rituals, and myths, among other things, are recorded.*

There is not one central sacred scripture like a "Bible of the Usui System." In relation to the rediscovery of the *Reiki Ryoho Hikkei*, the "Handbook of the Reiki Method of Healing" that dates back to Mikao Usui, there are sometimes tendencies to ascribe to it the status of a central scripture for the Usui System of Reiki. However, upon closer consideration it becomes clear that this handbook (cf. pg. 154 ff.) cannot fulfill these types of expectations since it ultimately has too little substance and leaves too many questions open.

- *A founding figure upon whom the religion is based.*

The Usui System of Reiki has a founding figure in Mikao Usui, whose name has even become part of the general term for the system (Usui System of Reiki) in the course of time. However, since Mikao Usui, as explained in detail in other places, hardly had a lasting, form-giving influence on the many different forms that have evolved from the system that he created, his work was more like the one of an establishing figure than of a founder. One characteristic of an establishing figure is that his work is less specific than that of a founder. While a founder usually defines the system that he has developed in all of its details, therefore bringing it into a clear, timeless form, the work of an establishing figure can be described as a person who prepares the ground so that something can develop.

- *An institution, meaning an organization, which has been created for practicing the respective religion.*
There is not a central institution that has been created for the practice of the Usui System of Reiki. However, there are institutions and/or organizations existing within the various forms of the Usui System that fulfill this purpose. For instance, the *Usui Shiki Ryoho* has the "Office of the Grandmaster (OGM)," as well as an association of Masters who teach this form, The Reiki Alliance.

- *Sacred places, meaning cult places and/or buildings, as well as holy days.*
The Usui System of Reiki does not have any holy places or holy days. However, with the publication of new information about the beginning times of the Usui System it has become well-known in recent years that Mikao Usui had what was probably a central, enlightening experience for the Usui System of Reiki on the sacred Japanese Mount Kurama near Kyoto. In addition, it has become common knowledge that there is a memorial stone erected in his honor at the Saihoji Temple in Tokyo. Some practitioners have since visited these places, sometimes with the attitude of making a connection with the original essence of the Usui System in this way. However, it would certainly be an exaggeration to give these places the status of holy places in relation to the Usui System.

Summary: Only certain portions of the Usui System of Reiki meet the main characteristics of a religion. So the Usui System can hardly be called a religion. Yet, it should be clear by now that the community of those who practice the Usui System definitely bears some of the traits of a religious community.

⌒⟶

The Usui System as a Microcosm

As this chapter shows, the Usui System of Reiki in its entirety is ultimately a "melting pot" of various spiritual forms and contents. At the same time, when we consider the aspects of esoteric disciplines together with the traits of religious communities, we have a microcosm that is virtually exemplary of the spiritual development of humanity as a whole.

Living spirituality in everyday life and in the world is important, also for practitioners of the Usui System of Reiki. The Dalai Lama has written the following about the task that the spiritual traditions fulfill in our modern age:

"I usually speak of two levels of spirituality. One kind of spirituality has to do with faith. The other is not necessarily religious faith; it simply has to do with having good human qualities, such as a sense of caring for one another, a sense of community, and a sense of responsibility. We can have a happy world without a religious government, but a happy world is not possible without good human qualities. So, within that context, spiritual traditions have an important role, which is to increase or extend basic human values and make a contribution for a better, more compassionate world."[8]

I am convinced that practitioners of the Usui System, as those who practice a spiritual tradition that is widespread throughout the world and whose practice consists of laying on hands—meaning personal attention—could contribute a great deal to this development.

10. Healing

Accepting the Paradox

The Usui System of Reiki is now well-known throughout the world as the "No. 1 Folk Healing Art." It is considered to be "a spiritual method of healing for everyone." In addition, doctors, nurses, physiotherapists, and members of other helping professions are also beginning to learn the Usui System of Reiki and/or work together with experienced practitioners of the system.

One of the first larger scientific studies on the effects of Reiki treatments was published in the spring of 2003 in the renowned American magazine *Alternative Therapies.*[1] One of the authors, the Reiki Master Pamela Miles, introduced the Usui System of Reiki to a number of major New York clinics.[2] There are already more than 100 hospitals in the USA in which Reiki treatments are offered.[3] The cooperation between Reiki practitioners and hospitals or clinics is also increasing in Europe, above all in Great Britain, Switzerland, and most recently also in Germany.

In addition to the majority of Reiki practitioners throughout the world who welcome this development, there are also some who are critical of it. They are afraid that the spiritual aspect of the Usui System could be lost in hospitals and that Reiki treatments may just be seen as a type of medical intervention. Pamela Miles responded in the following manner to this perspective in an interview published in *Reiki Magazine International:*

"I don't see how the spiritual aspect of Reiki can possibly be in danger—that's what Reiki is. Reiki is spirit and nothing can divest Reiki of spirituality. We all share Reiki from our own understanding, and those who practice come to know the spiritual foundation of

Reiki more deeply over time. Reiki meets people where they are and quietly connects them to their innate spirituality. In general, I'm not concerned about the way other people practice Reiki. There are things I don't agree with and don't support, but I do support people's right to practice Reiki as they know it. I have trust and conviction in Reiki. To me, nothing is more powerful than Reiki. Reiki can return spirituality to medicine."[4]

What is Healing?

"Bringing medicine back to a more natural condition is important," writes Deepak Chopra, M.D., the internationally renowned physician and Ayurveda expert. According to Chopra, "the basic unit of medicine is natural, after all—a person in trouble seeking help from someone who knows the cure. Leaving medical technology aside, this relationship will always be best when it is simplest and therefore most natural."[5]

An uncomplicated and natural relationship between the physician or healer and the patient—it appears, as the work of many successful physicians and healers shows, that this is actually the basis for true healing to take place. If we look at which accompanying circumstances are also important in addition to this for healing to occur, we can essentially summarize them in the following points:

The basic precondition for any type of healing appears to be that the person who needs healing seeks a doctor or healer on his own. People generally will only do this when there is a certain pressure from suffering, when a physical or emotional affliction takes on dimensions that they can no longer manage alone.

If an encounter occurs between the healer and the patient, it is the task of the healer to create a natural, relaxed situation. Above all, this involves paying attention to the patient, truly seeing him with his suffering, and accepting the state in which he initially finds himself.

In the healing treatment, the healer ultimately uses a specific method of healing that corresponds with his or her abilities in order to have an influence that is concrete and healing. The goal of the treatment is basically to trigger the self-healing powers of the patient.

One part of the work of the healer is to break the pride of the patient. In addition, he or she must also make it clear to the patient that he is personally responsible for breaking the bad habits and/or ways of thinking that are the cause of the affliction.

The patient must be willing to truly let himself be helped by the healer. This means that he must allow the healer to have power over him for a certain time. This can only occur on the basis of trust.

With the progressing of the healing process, the patient must develop a certain degree of devotion to his own healing. In any case, he must have the unrestricted desire to actually achieve healing. In addition, positive thinking, a loving attitude toward himself and other people, as well as general healing activities in everyday life are helpful.

In the Christian perspective, true healing is accompanied by the perception that we are ultimately not separate from God.

According to the teachings of Buddha, the process of healing is similar to that of spiritual development:

"Buddha frequently used disease and healing as a comparison for making various aspects of his teachings understandable. According to his teachings, every human being who has not achieved liberation, who is still subject to suffering, which brings the insatiable desire with it, can be considered 'sick.' The healing process is therefore similar to the process in which one achieves enlightenment."[6]

⌒

The Ultimate Truth

"With the evolution theory of Charles Darwin, the Christian Teachings finally had the origin mythos taken from them. The explanation monopoly of our origin belonged to the natural sciences from that time on."[7]

What this author has written about the effects of the evolution theory on the Christian origin mythos also applies in a similar way to the effects that the rediscovery of the information about the beginning period of the Usui System had on the legendary form of the history of the system. Through the rediscovery, a development was set in motion in which the explanations about the origin of the Usui System was no longer dominated by storytellers but by people who had researched the historical correlations and presented dates and facts.

However, this author is mistaken when he thinks that a mythos can simply be "taken" away from a religious community or its teachings as a result of a new theory (even if the theory is based on facts that appear to contradict the contents of the mythos). A mythos draws its power, and therefore its validity, not from the fact that its content can be proven but from the timeless truth of the described correlations that comes from deep within it. And these should not be taken "literally" but bear their truth "between the lines." Ultimately, a mythos is not an explanation but an illustration of the correlations.

That same approach applies to the legendary form of the history of the Usui System: It can also not be "taken" from the Reiki practitioners through the rediscovery of information about the beginning period of the Usui System. Just like a mythos, the legendary form of the history does not draw its power from the fact that its content can be proven but much more from the timeless truth within it, which can ultimately be found "between the lines."

The history of the Usui System of Reiki continues every day. All Reiki practitioners are a part of it. Some of the rediscovered information may become a part of the history of the system in time. However, the rediscovery, which was undertaken by Reiki practitioners after all, will itself become a part of the history of the system, integrating it into the sequence of events that create the core of the history. And, who knows: Perhaps the event of the rediscovery will be presented in exactly the same legendary way in the distant future as the beginnings of the history are today?

The history of the Usui System of Reiki is alive. It can never be static. The history consists of more than just dates and facts. It lives from the little episodes and the larger correlations, from the strands that can be varied, from "close-ups" that can be described as scenes. It lives from events that actually took place, as well as what has been "added" to them. It lives from the characters, the actions that they take, and from what develops out of them.

And: What would a story be if we could not constantly tell it in a new way?

Shortly after I finished the work on this book, I held a First Degree seminar. On Friday evening I told the legendary form of the history of the Usui System as beautifully as never before. It was absolutely still, the participants were moved as they listened, and I felt how the history took on a life of its own and had been awakened to a new life through my confrontation with it in the form of this book. The legend and the facts went hand in hand, the flow of the story was beautifully round, and all of the contradictions vanished in thin air.

Today, on Saturday during the lunch break, I sit alone in the seminar room and rest. I give myself Reiki and look at the little table upon which the photos of Mikao Usui, Dr. Hayashi, Hawayo Takata, and Phyllis Furumoto stand, each of them set in an exquisite frame, on a cloth embroidered with Buddhist symbols. Deep within myself, I am happy … I am happy about this moment, the coming afternoon, the evening at home, just for today …

Epilog
A Parable

Once there was a man who, after a long search in various parts of the world, found a way to re-establish the connection to the greater whole; this is what the people had lost over the course of time. He truly did great things for the people by awakening the inner forces within human beings in a moment of grace, as well as teaching them to train their minds and heal diseases. Yet, his greatest gift was that he not only taught others the way but also even transmitted to some of them the ability to also teach the way as he did. After this man died much too early, those who had received from him the ability to teach the way continued his work. In addition to a group that continued to teach the way like he had shown them, there was a man who began to teach the way in a somewhat different way on the basis of his own convictions and experiences. Since he was very successful in using it with people, he felt that it was justified.

One day, a woman came from a distant land and wanted to learn the way from him. After some initial difficulties, this woman became the man's best student and, shortly before his death, he designated her as his successor. The woman returned to her homeland and began teaching the way in these new surroundings. Even though she was capable of transmitting to others the ability to also teach the way, she waited a long time to do this. In the meantime, she simply taught others the way and helped people wherever she could. In the course of time, she also began teaching the way in a somewhat different manner on the basis of her own convictions and experiences. As she did this, she placed more value on healing diseases than training the mind. Shortly before her death, she began transmitting to others the ability to also teach the way. She died at an old age.

It now became evident that many people throughout the world felt touched by the way in which the woman taught it and also wanted to learn how to teach it. The granddaughter of the woman and others who had received from her the ability to teach the way decided to preserve this form and continued to teach the way as the woman had done. One of the other students of the woman, who had also received the ability to teach the way, now thought that she was the only one who had received the complete map for the way from the woman. Yet, since her experience of the way did not correspond with what the other students had received from the woman, she kept to herself and began teaching people the way by using the complete map. However, she later no longer called it the way but the path.

After more and more people had learned the way and many of them had received the ability to also teach the way, many new varieties of the way, most of which were further developments, connections of the way with other ways, sometimes even with streets, alleys, or tracks. In some cases, the way even turned into a type of trail since many of those who had received the ability to teach the way had not been careful and given it enough care. After the way had spread throughout the earth, there was an increased interest in the man who had once created the way. Since it had not been very long since his death, some curious people began to do research. In the process, they ultimately discovered the descendents of those who once had learned the path directly from the man who created the way.

These descendents still taught the way in the same manner as their ancestors had shown them. However, they were not pleased about the entire development and felt overwhelmed by it. As a result, they kept very much to themselves. Furthermore, some people were found who, in addition to the woman, had learned the way from the man who had begun to teach it in a somewhat different manner. Ultimately, it was discovered that the manner in which the way was originally taught placed just as much importance on training the mind as healing diseases. As a result, some people started to orient themselves more upon what had originally been taught and no longer upon what had developed over time. On the other hand, quite a large group saw no reason to do this because they did not feel that something was missing. Some people out of this group had long ago integrated the training of the mind in a different manner into their practice of the way. And then there were others who did not think that mind training was very important at all.

In addition to those who now shifted their orientation to what had been originally taught and those who continued to be satisfied with what had developed over time, there were those who increasingly asked the question: Where does the way lead? They frequently received answers that caused them to leave the outer form of the way behind them and completely dedicate themselves to the essence of the way from that point on. In the process, it was not important for them that they lost every kind of external frame of reference. And then there were those who increasingly asked the question: Where does the way come from? They primarily found answers that caused them to place more emphasis on the source from which the man had developed the way than what the man had created. In view of the new findings that showed a very different, much larger way as the basis for creating the way, they now found the form of the way created by the man to be too limited. Yet, they also had to admit that without the work of the man and the form of the way that he had created, they would never have found the larger way that was its basis because it had been lost to the people before the man had rediscovered parts of it.

However, the majority of the people who took the way and taught it continued to follow the way in its simple form, as the woman developed it. Time passed and now people became aware of the way who actually did not follow any ways at all. After they became more familiar with the way, they began to classify the various forms of manifestation of the way according to whether they were more of a "footpath" or a "roadway." These people promised themselves a greater consciousness for people involved with the way since, after it had spread around the world, it had received a special significance for all people and concerned everyone as a result. The people who followed the way received one or the other insight in response to this. Yet, deep within themselves they still knew that such classifications were ultimately not very important. According to the perceptions of many people who had taken the way to its end, what ultimately counted was just one thing: how the person takes the way.

Appendix

Little Dictionary of Reiki

Terms from A to Z

Affirmation

Affirmations are constructive, life-encouraging sentences that are used on the mental level through frequent repetition for purposes such as increasing health and well-being. In the Usui System of Reiki, affirmations may be used in the mental treatment, among other areas. / *cf.: Mental Treatment*

Alliance

see: The Reiki Alliance

Animals

Many practitioners of the Usui System also treat animals with Reiki, such as their pets, animals on farms, or just simply animals that show them that they would like to receive Reiki. These are frequently dogs, cats, horses, or even birds. In general, animals are very uncomplicated in dealing with Reiki. They usually have a fine sense for energies and immediately know intuitively that someone wants to give them Reiki. When animals want to receive Reiki, they usually approach us on their own, clearly showing where they would like to receive the Reiki. They allow themselves to be treated and then get up and leave when they have had enough.

Application

Some practitioners speak of a "Reiki application" when they give Reiki. Others call it a "Reiki treatment." The various terms are accompanied by different opinions as to the basic nature of giving Reiki. However, the use of specific terms may also have legal grounds.

Aromatherapy

This is a form of healing treatment with aromatic substances, usually in the form of essential oils. The most widespread application is vaporizing the oils, mixed with water, in a fragrance lamp. Some practitioners of the Usui System use essential oils in combination with Reiki. An example of this is using the appropriate essential oil in a fragrance lamp, which dissipates it throughout the room, for example during a Reiki treatment.

Attunement

see: Initiation

Aura

Multi-layered, invisible, subtle energy body that surrounds the physical body. In the Usui System of Reiki, some practitioners use the technique of "stroking the aura." This involves the practitioner using both hands to slowly stroke along the body of the person receiving treatment from the head to the feet at the beginning and end of a treatment, usually three times, at a distance of about 8-20 inches. Some practitioners of the Usui System also give Reiki, as they say, directly into the aura of the person receiving treatment. To do this, they do not place their hands on the body but keep them floating at a small distance from the physical body.

Aura-Soma

Aura-Soma is a holistic healing method that was founded in the 1980s by Vicky Wall of England. The Aura-Soma system consists of colorful, fragrant oils and essences that are made from plant extracts and gemstone energies. They are used by applying them to the skin or fanning them into the aura. Some practitioners of the Usui System use the Aura-Soma essences in combination with Reiki. The Pomanders and Quintessences are best suited for this purpose. For example, they can be used—in as far as they are appropriate for the theme at hand—by fanning them into the aura of the client before or after a treatment. / see pg. 191.

Authentic Reiki®

This is one of the terms for The Radiance Technique®, whose teachings and practice go back to Dr. Barbara Ray. / *cf.: The Radiance Technique®* / see pg. 96.

Bach Flowers

This is a natural method of healing based on the flower essences developed by Dr. Edward Bach. The total of 38 Bach Flower essences are suited for the treatment of chronic diseases, as well as the treatment of acute conditions such as situations of psychological stress. Like Reiki, they are well-suited for self-treatment. Some practitioners of the Usui System use the Bach Flower essences in combination with Reiki. Anyone who would like to work on a specific emotional theme can take the respective essence orally or apply it to the corresponding part of the body. This is also possible directly before a Reiki treatment, which can more intensely call into consciousness a specific topic. Furthermore, the hands can be sprinkled with the corresponding essence directly before giving Reiki so that Reiki continually flows through the "filter" of this Bach Flower essence, this emotional theme, during the treatment. / See pg. 184.

Back Treatment

This is part of the full-body treatment with Reiki. A full-body treatment generally concludes with the back treatment. In the various forms of the Usui System, about five to seven basic positions are generally used for treating the back, as well as some secondary positions for the treatment of specific problem areas such as the spinal column or back of the neck. / cf.: *Full-Body Treatment, Hand Positions*

Byosen

During the lifetime of Mikao Usui and Dr. Hayashi, the technique of *byosen* was the most important foundation for the treatment with Reiki. *Byosen* means something like the "vibration of the disease." The technique of *byosen* involves finding the source of the disease vibration in the body of the person to be treated and leaving the hands there until the vibration changes or dissolves. *Byosen* can be found where the cause of the disease is located. This does not always have to be where the pain or a symptom manifests. During the lifetime of Mikao Usui and Dr. Hayashi, only those who had attained a certain sense of confidence in the technique of *byosen* were allowed to learn the Second Degree, *Okuden*. / see pg. 45.

Certificate

The majority of Reiki Masters and Teachers fill out a corresponding certificate for their students as they attain each of the degrees of the system. The certificates used vary in form and content. They usually contain the name of the student, the place and date of the initiation, as well as the name of the initiating Master/Teacher. The certificates frequently include the personal stamp of the Master/Teacher. If the Master/Teacher is a member of a Reiki (Teacher) association, the signed certificate may also include the stamp of the respective association. In addition, the certificate may have golden seals and/or colored ribbons.

Chakras

These are the energy centers that are located in the subtle body of a human being. The word chakra comes from the Sanskrit language and means something like "wheel." The many, sometimes very different teachings about the chakras generally recognize seven major chakras. According to the ancient Hindu scriptures, there are a total of 88,000 chakras in the subtle body of a human being. Some practitioners of the Usui System use Reiki in combination with the chakra work. A widespread approach is the so-called chakra-balancing in which each of the seven major chakras are treated with Reiki, one after the other. In this approach, either each chakra is treated with both hands at the same time from above to below, for example (seven positions) or two chakras are treated simultaneously with one hand on each of them. For example: the Root and the Crown Chakras at the same time, then the Sacral Chakra and the Third Eye at the same time, then the Solar-Plexus Chakra and the Throat Chakra at the same time, and then finishing with the Heart Chakra using both hands at the same time (four positions). / See pg. 206 ff.

Channel

Practitioners of the Usui System frequently call themselves a "channel" for the universal life energy. It can also be important for the personal development of practitioners to not just see themselves as a "channel" in the use of Reiki but also be aware that with intensified, disciplined practice of the system it becomes increasingly possible to embody the universal life energy within the being of the individual person.

Channeling

During a channeling session, a psychic person, also called a medium, imparts information or messages to the people who are listening or later reads a record of the session. Usually a group of people come together for a channeling session, during which a medium channels messages or information from spiritual entities to those present. / See pg. 225 ff.

Cleansing Phase

Books about the Usui System frequently state that a three-week cleansing phase takes place in the body of the initiate directly after the initiation into the First Degree. This may be the experience of some practitioners of the system. However, the cleansing phase that begins with the initiation into the First Degree basically cannot be limited to the three weeks after the First Degree seminar. Instead, the regular practice of the system in the form of daily self-treatment is accompanied by a continual cleansing on the physical and spiritual level that is sometimes more and sometimes less in the foreground. Yet, it will take place continually as long as the initiate practices in a serious and regular manner.

Color Therapy

Color therapy is considered to be one of the oldest treatment methods of humanity. In the beginning, the starting point was in the healing power of the sunlight, which was especially valued by the Egyptians, as well as by the Mayans and the Aztecs. Later, the perception that individual colors have specific effects was generally accepted. The use of colors for healing purposes began shortly thereafter. Today there are various methods that range from color-radiation devices to colored glasses and color baths, color acupuncture, and color meditations. The Lüscher Color Test, developed by Professor Dr. Max Lüscher has become well-known and is used throughout the world by medical professionals and psychologists. In esotericism, the colors have a great symbolic significance. They are generally intended to help achieve a specific frequency or mood. However, there is no uniform scheme for classifying them, which means that they are very different depending upon the spiritual direction, discipline, or school. Some practitioners use methods of color therapy in combination with Reiki. When decorating their treatment rooms, many practitioners make sure that the predominate colors support the healing process in accordance with the respectively represented psychological or spiritual direction.

Contraindication

This is the term for circumstances in which the use of an essentially effective healing treatment is prohibited. Reiki practitioners are divided in their opinions as to what can represent contraindication in relation to Reiki treatments. While some believe that there definitely are contraindications (and also give examples of treatments that they have experienced in which problems repeatedly occurred under the same, specific circumstances), others express the viewpoint that there can be no contraindications in relation to Reiki treatments (and base this opinion on the fact that they have never experienced repeated problems in treatments under the same, specific circumstances, even not in such circumstances that others call contraindications such as "the person receiving treatment was anesthetized" or "the person receiving treatment has a heart pacemaker.")

Death Accompaniment

In addition to healing diseases of a physical and spiritual nature, as well as generally strengthening the life forces, the accompaniment of the dying is also an area of application for Reiki practitioners.

Distant Healing

This term is usually used as a synonym for the technique of distant treatment. / *cf.: Distant Treatment, Distant Reiki*

Distant-Healing Symbol

This term is used for the third symbol of the Second Degree, which enables the initiate to give distant treatments with Reiki. / *cf.: Distant Reiki, Power Symbol, Master Symbol, Mental-Healing Symbol, Symbols*

Distant Initiation

This is a form of initiation in which a Reiki Master or teacher says that he or she performs the corresponding initiation without the physical presence of the individual who is intended to receive it. Even if the possibility of a successfully completed distant initiation cannot be completely dismissed if it is performed by a very experienced person who is highly developed in terms of spirituality, this procedure appears to be so far removed from any of the traditional forms of teachings in the Usui System that the majority of all Reiki Masters and teachers agree that this form of initiation has very little in common with the Usui System of Reiki.

Distant Reiki

This term is generally used among practitioners of the Usui System for the sending of Reiki per distant treatment.

Distant Treatment

This is a technique of the Second Degree that makes it possible for the initiate to send Reiki over a distance. / *cf.: Distant-Healing Symbol, Distant Reiki, Emergency Chains, Reiki Box*

Emergency Chains

Reiki practitioners who are initiated into at least the Second Reiki Degree frequently join together into so-called "emergency chains." In the case of a personal crisis, an accident, or other difficult situations concerning the people participating in the "emergency chain" or their loved ones, the chain is activated. Each person calls another in a previously established order with the goal of informing as many of the participating people as possible of the critical situation and being able to send the afflicted person one or more distant treatments with Reiki. / *cf.: Distant Treatment, Second Degree*

Energy Exchange

A generally common term among Reiki Masters and teachers, as well as practitioners, for the concept that they receive something from the seminar participants and/or clients in exchange for initiations into the various degrees of the Usui System of Reiki, as well as the corresponding seminars and Reiki treatments. In most cases, this refers to money, especially for Reiki seminars. However, this may also be other things or services such as an invitation for a meal, concert tickets, help with the garden work, especially in exchange for treatments. The receipt of money or another service on the part of the Reiki Master/Teacher and practitioners is seen as an exchange for the energy that they use to give the Reiki seminars and/or treatments, but not as payment for the universal life energy of Reiki, which obviously cannot be paid for. Many practitioners share the opinion that an energy exchange is absolutely necessary if genuine healing is to take place. Among other things, this approach is based upon the concept that only those who also give something actually value what they receive. Many Reiki Masters and teachers insist that a specific amount of money is paid in exchange by the participants for involvement in the Reiki seminars so that the initiations can unfold their full effect. On the other hand, a few Reiki Masters and teacher dispense entirely with payment in a certain amount and offer initiations and treatments on a donation basis. / cf. pg. 180.

Exchange Meeting

Many Reiki Masters and teachers organize Reiki-exchange meetings on a regular basis. These take place once a month or every two weeks, for example, and make it possible for the students to stay in contact with the Master/Teacher. During the exchange meeting, students generally have the possibility of directing questions to the teacher, engage in an exchange with each other, and participate in a group treatment. / *cf.: Group Treatment*

First Degree

The First Degree of the Usui System of Reiki is usually taught within the framework of a two- or three-day seminar. The participants generally receive four initiations and practice the hand positions for self-treatment and the treatment of others with Reiki. They listen to the history of the Usui System and become familiar with the five Reiki Principles. Important topics related to Reiki are addressed and questions are answered. After the conclusion of the seminar, the participants are able to transmit the universal life energy of

Reiki to themselves and others through the laying-on of hands. / *cf.: Initiation, Second Degree, Third Degree*

First Symbol

see: Power Symbol

Foot Initiations

Some Reiki Masters and teachers also perform the so-called "foot initiations" within the scope of the usual initiation rituals. The intention, according to the basic idea of this initiation practice, is to increase the grounding of the person who is being initiated. According to everything that we know today, neither Mikao Usui nor Dr. Hayashi nor Hawayo Takata performed "foot initiations." So this initiation practice is most likely based upon the work of Gerda E. Drescher, the founder of Rei-Ki Balancing®. However, in relation to her new development, she did not refer to "foot initiations" but performing energetic attunements on the feet or additional foot openings. / See pg. 112.

Full-Body Treatment

This form of the treatment with Reiki covers the entire body. The person who is giving himself or herself the treatment or a second individual receiving the treatment is usually in a prone position. A complete full-body treatment lasts about 60 to 90 minutes. It generally includes the treatment of the head, the front side of the body, and the back side of the body. According to the direction of the Usui System, the treatment of the legs, the feet, and the arms may also be part of the full-body treatment. While most forms of the Usui System have established sequences of hand positions for the full-body treatment, both for the self-treatment and the treatment of others, some practitioners prefer to trust their own intuition in terms of the positions of their hands. / *cf.: Hand Positions, Head Treatment, Back Treatment*

Gassho Posture

Placing the palms of the hands together and holding them in front of the heart with the fingers pointing upward. / See pg. 152.

Gemstones

In all known cultures, gemstones have always been used as jewelry and for healing purposes. The stones are worn on the body or placed on it with this intention. Some practitioners of the Usui System use gemstones in combination with Reiki. It is possible to work with a great variety of stones in this way. For example, seven stones of the same type—such as rose quartz—are placed on the seven major chakras while Reiki is given. Another possibility is including quartz crystals in the Reiki application: Crystals have a clarifying, cleansing effect. It is said that Mikao Usui also worked with gemstones. He apparently sometimes charged crystal balls with Reiki, which were then laid directly on the afflicted body parts of the person to be treated with Reiki. / See pg. 197.

Gendai Reiki Ho

Method of practicing Reiki that was developed by the Japanese Reiki Teacher Hiroshi Doi on the basis of his many experiences with a great variety of Reiki systems. Doi explains that he has combined "Western and Japanese traditional methods" with each other. / See pg. 166.

Grand Master

There is no Grand Master that heads the entire Usui System of Reiki such as the Dalai Lama of Tibetan Buddhism. Since the death of Mikao Usui, there is no longer anyone who is considered to be the sole authority by the practitioners of all the existing forms and styles of the Usui System. In some forms of the Usui System, there is now the title of the Grand Master, but other forms of the Usui System do not have such a title. If such a title exists, it is reserved for one individual person. For example, Phyllis Furumoto currently bears the title of the Grand Master in *Usui Shiki Ryoho,* which means that she holds the spiritual lineage of this system and represents an authority figure for the practitioners of this system. She received the title by becoming the successor of her grandmother, Hawayo Takata, who was called the "Grand Master" by her students during the last years of her life. This is probably also the origin of this title within the Usui System of Reiki. During the lifetimes of Mikao Usui and Dr. Hayashi, the title of Grand Master apparently did not exist. In recent times, some "independent Masters" have begun to initiate other Masters into the so-called "Grand Master Degree." Within this context, the term of "Grand Master" is understood as a type of expanded degree instead of a special title; this is generally the highest degree that can be achieved within the respective practice. However, this does not mean that the person given the name of "Grand Master" in this way represents an authority for all those involved in the respective practice. / *cf.: Spiritual Lineage*

Group Treatment

This is a form of the treatment with Reiki in which several practitioners give a person Reiki at the same time. During a group treatment, between three and eight practitioners generally form a group. Each of the participants usually receives treatment from all of the others simultaneously for a certain amount of time, such as ten or twenty minutes. / *cf.: Exchange Meeting*

Hand Positions

The hands are placed directly on the body during a Reiki treatment. Although there is an established sequence of hand positions in most forms of the Usui System for self-treatment and the treatment of other persons, some practitioners prefer to trust their own intuition in terms of their hand positions during treatments. In addition to the standard positions, such as the eight basic positions for self-treatment and the 14 basic positions for the treatment of another person, a large number of special positions for the treatment of

291

specific physical and emotional problems are now well-known and even fill entire books. The basic rule for all forms of standard treatment is that every hand position is held from about three to five minutes. Even Mikao Usui and Dr. Hayashi created so-called "Treatment Plans" that contained many hand positions, especially for the treatment of specific diseases. / *cf.: Full-Body Treatment, Head Treatment, Back Treatment* / See pg. 69 f., pg. 156 ff.

Hatsureiho
A form of meditation that probably dates back to Mikao Usui. It serves to intensify the general flow of the Reiki energy. *Hatsu* means something like "starting up" or "stimulating," *rei* is the "rei" of Reiki, and *ho* means method. Mikao Usui reportedly recommended to his students that they practice *Hatsureiho* in the morning and evening of every day. / See pg. 22.

Head Treatment
This is part of the full-body treatment with Reiki. A full-body treatment generally begins with the head treatment. In the various forms of the Usui System, each has about three to five well-known basic positions for the treatment of the head, as well as some secondary positions for treating specific problem areas such as the mouth or throat. / *cf.: Full-Body Treatment, Hand Positions*

History
The history of the Usui System of Reiki is part of the teachings of the system. It is usually told by the Reiki Master and/or teacher in every First Degree seminar. / See pg. 9 ff., pg. 265, pg. 272 ff.

Independent Masters
This is a colloquial term for the Reiki Masters and teachers who do not feel that they belong to any specific form of the Usui System of Reiki in their practice and teaching. / See pg. 177 ff.

Individual Treatment

In this form of treatment with Reiki, one practitioner treats one other person. / *cf.: Group Treatment, Self-Treatment*

Initiation

In the Usui System of Reiki, this is the ceremony or ritual that the Reiki Master or teacher does for the students. The initiation into the First Degree generally includes four ceremonies (in some styles of the Usui System there are also fewer), which together are considered the "initiation into the First Degree." This enables the students to transmit the universal life energy of Reiki through the laying-on of hands on themselves and others. The initiation into the Second Degree generally includes one ceremony (in some styles of the Usui System there are also more). This enables the students to use the three symbols of the Second Degree for intensifying the flow of Reiki, for the mental treatment, and for the distant treatment. The initiation into the Master Degree (also called the Third Degree) generally includes one ceremony. This enables the initiated person to initiate others in turn into the First Degree, the Second Degree, and the Third Degree. It is generally expected that a newly initiated Master/Teacher only begin with the training of other Masters/Teachers after a corresponding waiting period of several years in order to have sufficient experiences in the activities of a Master/Teacher. The course of the ceremonies, which consist of the initiations into the various degrees, are transmitted from Master/Teacher to Master/Teacher. The initiation is sometimes also called attunement or activation. / *cf.: First Degree, Second Degree, Third Degree*

Initiation Lineage

see: Lineage

Jikiden Reiki

This form of Reiki was developed by the Japanese Reiki Teacher Chiyoko Yamaguchi on the basis of her experiences with the teachings of Dr. Hayashi. Since the death of Chiyoko Yamaguchi in 2003, her son, Tadao Yamaguchi, has continued her life work. / See pg. 163.

Karuna Reiki®

Established by William Lee Rand and based on the Usui System of Reiki, this new form of working with the universal life energy is directed exclusively at Reiki Teachers and/or Masters. This system is based on channeled information. / *cf.: Channeling* / See pg. 135 ff.

Ki

This is the name for one of the two characters that come together to form the term "Reiki." The Japanese word *Ki* can be translated in a number of different ways. A common translation into English is "life energy." The word *Ki* is also part of the names of other Far-Eastern disciplines that work with the life energy such as "Aikido," "Tai Chi, and "Qi Gong." It is sometimes expressed with a different spelling in these terms, such as Qi or Chi, but still means the same thing. Other meanings for this word that can be interpreted in many ways are "spirit," "heart," "soul," "intention," "mood," and "temperament." / *cf.: Rei, Reiki*

Licensing

During the 1990s, there were incidents within the world-wide Reiki scene that caused the Lineage Bearer of the *Usui Shiki Ryoho*, Phyllis Furumoto, to want to have the terms "Reiki" and "Usui Shiki Ryoho" protected throughout the world as trademarks. After one of the Reiki Masters who she had initiated in Germany had the Reiki character legally registered as a trademark in his name and had already begun to prohibit the use of the Japanese character and the words "Reiki" by other Reiki Masters and teachers in the German-language region who did not teach what he considered to be the true, traditional Usui System, Phyllis Furumoto saw herself compelled to prevent similar developments in other countries by attempting to have the corresponding terms and characters protected under her name. However, it soon became clear that the expressions "Reiki" and "Usui Shiki Ryoho" could not be protected in most countries. Since her action did not receive the support of a majority within the respective Reiki Master community, the plan, which included a system of granting licenses with respect to the *Usui Shiki Ryoho,* was dropped. In the countries in which it was possible to protect the corresponding expressions, this was done with the result that they now can also be freely used by anyone in these countries. / *cf.: Usui Shiki Ryoho*

Lineage

In the Usui System of Reiki, the term "lineage" describes the line of the Masters and/or Teachers through whom the Usui System of Reiki has come to a person beginning with Mikao Usui, up to the Master/Teacher from whom the initiation has been received. Every person who has been initiated into Reiki has a lineage, no matter what degree he or she has. Here are two examples of this: 1. Mr. X has received the initiation into the First Degree from Master Y, who was initiated as a Master by Hawayo Takata. His lineage is: Mikao Usui—Dr. Chujiro Hayashi—Hawayo Takata—Master Y / 2. Ms. Z has received the initiation into the Master Degree from Master Y. Her lineage consists of: Mikao Usui—Dr. Chujiro Hayashi—Hawayo Takata—Master Y. If Ms. Z now does initiations, then the people that she has initiated are in this lineage: Mikao Usui—Dr. Chujiro Hayashi—Hawayo Takata—Master Y—Master Z. The lineage, also called the initiation lineage, characterizes the "energetic origin." Not only in the Usui System of Reiki, but also in other spiritual traditions such as Buddhism, the lineage through which a person has received a teaching is considered important. The terms "lineage" or "initiation lineage" are not identical with the "spiritual lineage." / *cf.: Spiritual Lineage*

Mantras

Syllables or entire sequences of syllables that are filled with a spiritual meaning or a "magical power." Within the Reiki scene, there is no agreement on whether the terms for the three symbols of the Second Degree, as well as for the so-called Master Symbol, can be called mantras or whether these are simply terms that have no mantra-like effect in the original sense of the word. / See pg. 220.

Master

This is the short form used in the Usui System of Reiki for "Reiki Master." / *cf.: Third Degree, Reiki Teacher, Reiki Master, Reiki Master/Teacher*

Master Candidate

In some forms of the Usui System, this is the term for someone who is taking the training to become a Reiki Master. / *cf.: Master Training, Reiki Master*

Master Degree

This is a term for the Third Degree or sometimes for the first level of the Third Degree. / *cf.: Third Degree, Teacher Degree, Reiki Master*

Master Symbol

This is the name of the so-called symbol that is received during the initiation into the Master Degree. However, in the more precise sense of the word, this is not a symbol but Japanese characters and their terms that together result in a sentence. By way of contrast, all three symbols of the Second Degree are symbols in the actual sense of the word and not Japanese characters (the Distant-Healing Symbol also does not consist of individual characters but is composed of the parts of various characters). / *cf.: Symbols*

Master/Teacher

In the Usui System of Reiki, this is the short form for "Reiki Master/Teacher." / *cf.: Third Degree, Reiki Teacher, Reiki Master, Reiki Master/Teacher*

Master Training

In the training to become a Master, the students, who are sometimes called "Master Candidates," go through an apprenticeship in which they remain in close connection with the initiating Master. According to the style, the training to become a Master may last from several months to a number of years. The training should be started at a minimum of two to three years after receipt of the First Degree. After completion of the Master training and receipt of the related initiation, the initiate is capable of initiating other people into the First, Second, and Third Degree. It is usually expected that a newly initiated Master will only begin with the training of other Masters after a corresponding waiting period of several years. This time is necessary for them to have sufficient experience in the activities of a Master. There are currently no general guidelines for the training to become a Master. In terms of the content of the training, the initiating Master generally orients himself or herself upon the contents of his own training period and/or what is considered customary within the form of the Usui System that he or she practices. / Notes: In the styles of the Usui System that have a separation between the Master Degree and the Teacher Degree, the training to become a teacher generally corresponds with the training to become a Master as described here. In these styles, the receipt of the Master Degree consists solely of the initiation into the Master Degree and the transmission of the so-called Master Symbol. In the following time period, the training to become a teacher can take place, which is the training to enable a person to transmit the system to someone else; but this is not a must. On the other hand, in the forms of the Usui System in which there is no separation between the Master Degree and the Teacher Degree, the initiation into the Master Degree and the transmission of the so-called Master Symbol only takes place at the conclusion of the Master training after the successful training to enable the person to transmit the system to others. / *cf.: Third Degree, Master Candidate, Master Symbol, Reiki Master, Reiki Teacher*

Meditation

This is a general term for various forms of contemplation and/or the expansion of consciousness. In the process, the mind, the emotions, and the body come to complete rest. Some Reiki practitioners connect their practice of the Usui System with meditative practices or do a meditative practice in addition to the Usui System. Forms of meditation that date back to Mikao Usui include the *Hatsureiho* Meditation and the *Gassho* Meditation. / *cf.: Gassho Posture, Hatsureiho* / See pg. 152, pg. 22.

Meiji Emperor

The Meiji Emperor was generally a very popular emperor in Japan. He ruled the land during an unusually long period of 45 years, from 1868-1912, which was also during a large portion of Mikao Usui's lifetime. The term "Meiji" means something like "enlightened government" and describes the nature of this period of rulership under this Emperor, under whom a general enlightenment and opening came to the country. The Meiji Emperor reportedly wrote more than 100,000 poems during his lifetime. Like many other Japanese, Mikao Usui felt a high esteem for the Meiji Emperor and selected 125 of his poems that then played an important role in his teachings. Under Usui's direction, they were recited together, and he recommended that his students learn them as food for the mind. / See pg. 31.

Mental-Healing Symbol
This term is used for the second symbol of the Second Degree, which enables the initiate to give mental treatments. / *cf.: Mental Treatment, Power Symbol, Symbols*

Mental Treatment
This is one of the techniques of the Second Degree, which enables a deeper form of the treatment with Reiki. / *cf.: Mental-Healing Symbol*

Money
See: Energy Exchange

Mount Kurama
This is considered to be a sacred mountain in Japan and has many legends related to it. Mount Kurama is home to numerous temples of various spiritual traditions. It is located close to Kyoto and seen as the "spiritual heart of Japan." Mount Kurama is 570 meters high. Mikao Usui reportedly received the knowledge of Reiki during his 21-day fasting period while in deep meditation on Mount Kurama.

Okuden
This is the Japanese word for the Second Reiki Degree. It means something like "the deepest or last teaching." / *cf.: Shinpiden, Shoden* / See pg. 30, pg. 42.

Osho Neo-Reiki
A system developed by the German Reiki Master Himani H. Gerber in the circle of the Indian Master Osho (formerly Bhagwan) that is based on the Usui System of Reiki according to Hawayo Takata. / See pg. 119.

299

Plants

In addition to people and animals, many practitioners of the Usui System also treat plants with Reiki, including their houseplants or flowers and plants, vegetables, and trees growing in the great outdoors. For example, potted plants can be treated by holding the pot with both hands (here Reiki flows through the pot to the roots of the plant) or by treating the twigs and leaves directly or at a close distance. Trees can be actually "hugged" while giving them Reiki. There are no limits to the imagination when treating plants, flowers, vegetables, and trees.

Power Symbol

This is a term for the first symbol of the Second Degree, which enables the initiate to intensify the flow of Reiki. In addition, the first symbol can also be used in relation to the second and third symbol of the Second Degree. / *cf.: Distant-Healing Symbol, Mental-Healing Symbol, Symbols*

Principles

The five Reiki Principles are components of the teachings of the Usui System. Many different formulations of the principles have developed over time. One form that dates back to Mikao Usui: "Just for today, don't get angry. Don't worry. Show appreciation. Work hard. Be kind to others." / See pg. 21, pg. 67, pg. 95, pg. 263.

Radiance Technique

See: The Radiance Technique®

Rainbow Reiki

Developed by the German Reiki Master Walter Lübeck and based on the Usui System of Reiki according to Takata, *Rainbow Reiki* integrates the traditional Japanese methods, the work with the Inner Child, the Higher Self and angels, the essence technique,

KarmaClearing, systematic chakra work, and meditation, among other things. / See pg. 103.

Rei

This is the name for one of the two characters that form the term "Reiki." However, the Japanese expression *Rei* can be translated in a number of ways. A common translation into English is "universal." Other meanings of the term are "spiritual," "sacred," "the hidden power," or "the concealed meaning." / *cf.*: *Ki, Reiki*

Reiju Energy Transmission

This is a form of energy transmission that dates back to Mikao Usui. It is probably the original form of the initiation. Rei is the *"rei"* of Reiki, and *"ju"* means the "transmission from the teacher to the student." During Usui's lifetime, there was apparently just one initiation for those learning the First Degree, a "transmission of the *rei.*" But Usui constantly emphasized that it was important to participate in the regularly occurring student meetings in which there were additional Reiju energy transmissions. / See pg. 25.

Reiki

This word means "universal life energy" in Japanese. In addition to this customary translation into English, there are many other opportunities for translating the term and/or discovering its more profound meaning. Most practitioners of the Usui System use the term "Reiki" as a synonym for the practice of the Usui System. For example, a statement like "I do Reiki" means that the respective person transmits the universal life energy of Reiki by the laying-on of hands, which is possible after he or she has been initiated into the First Degree of the Usui System. / *cf.*: *Ki, Rei* / Also see: *"The Meaning of the Reiki Character"* by Walter Lübeck in: *The Spirit of Reiki*, Lotus Press.

Reiki Alliance
See: The Reiki Alliance

Reiki Association
See: The Reiki Association

Rei-Ki-Balancing®
A method established by the German Reiki Master Gerda E. Drescher that is based upon the Usui System of Reiki and focuses on grounding work. Energetic attunements on the feet play an important role in this approach. Since the death of Gerda E. Drescher in 2003, her work is being carried on by her husband, Edwin Zimmerli. / See pg. 112.

Reiki Box
This term is used by some practitioners of the Usui System for a little box in which to place slips of paper with personal wishes and/or positive affirmations. Afterward, Reiki is sent to the "Reiki Box" at regular intervals by the laying-on of hands or distant treatments with the goal of achieving fulfillment for the respective wishes and affirmations. / cf.: *Distant Treatment*

Reiki Jin Kei Do
This is a Reiki style whose spiritual lineage leads from Dr. Hayashi to the Venerable Takeuchi and the Venerable Seiji Takamori to the current lineage holder, Dr. Ranga Premaratna. The latter began spreading the Usui System imparted to him through the lineage of Takamori, as well as additional teachings based on Takamori's studies of Vajrayana Yoga, under the name of *Reiki Jin Kei Do*. / See pg. 124.

Reiki Magazines
The German-language *Reiki Magazin* was founded in 1997 by Jürgen Kindler and is still published quarterly in Germany, Austria, and Switzerland. There are or have been *Reiki Magazines*

in the following countries (listed chronologically according to the year of their founding here). In Switzerland: *Reiki Info* (in German, 1994-2000), *Info Reiki* (in French, 1996-1999); in Holland/Belgium: *Reiki Magazine* Nederland/België (in Dutch, since 1997); worldwide: *Reiki Magazine International* (in English, since 1999); in Argentina: *Reiki—Usui Shiki Ryoho* (in Spanish, 2000-2004); in the USA: *Reiki News Magazine* (in English, since 2002); in Brazil: *Via Reiki* (in Portuguese, since 2002); in Italy: *Reiki Magazine Italia* (in Italian, 2003-2004); in France: *Reiki Do Info* (in French, since 2004).

Reiki Master

In some styles of the Usui System, the term "Reiki Master" refers to someone who is initiated into the Third Degree and is therefore entitled to hold Reiki seminars. In other styles of the Usui System in which the Third Degree is divided into two levels, the term "Reiki Master" describes someone who has been initiated into the first level of the Third Degree, frequently called "3A" and has therefore only received the initiation into the Third Degree. However, this does not entitle him or her to also teach the Usui System (while someone who has also attained the second level of the Third Degree, which is frequently called "3B," is given the name of "Reiki Teacher" since he or she is entitled to teach the Usui System). In other styles of the Usui System, the term "Reiki Master" is not used at all. Even during Mikao Usui's lifetime, the term "Reiki Master" was apparently unknown. Only after Dr. Hayashi taught the Usui System of Reiki on Hawaii shortly before his death and had named Hawayo Takata as his successor, the term "Reiki Master" entered into the language of the Usui System. Above all, this was probably because the English language became necessary from that time on to describe the system. In the certificate signed by a notary public that Dr. Hayashi had prepared for Mrs. Takata and presented to her in 1938 on Hawaii, he speaks of both himself and Hawayo Takata as a "Reiki Master." / *cf.: Third Degree, Reiki Master, Reiki Master/Teacher*

Reiki Master/Teacher

This term combines the words "Reiki Master" and "Reiki Teacher" into one phrase. In those styles of the Usui System in which the Third Degree is divided into two levels, the term "Reiki Master/ Teacher" refers to someone who has attained both levels of the Third Degree. / *cf.: Third Degree, Reiki Teacher, Reiki Master*

Reiki Network

see: The Reiki Network

Reiki Outreach International

This is an internationally active Reiki organization with the goal of networking the energy of many Reiki practitioners in order to change difficult world situations such as wars, violence, nature catastrophes, and epidemics for the highest good of all. This generally occurs through distant treatments with Reiki. Reiki Outreach International (R.O.I.) currently has about 2,000 members throughout the world. / *cf.: Distant Treatment, Emergency Chains*

Reiki Ryoho

According to the inscription on the memorial stone for Mikao Usui, this is the original name of the method of healing that he established. *"Reiki"* means "the universal life energy," *"ryo"* means something like "healing", and *"ho"* means method. So the name *Reiki Ryoho* literally means something like the "Reiki Healing Method."

Reiki Shower

This term describes a technique intended to stimulate the flow of Reiki in the body. It is done by the Reiki practitioner visualizing a shower above his or her own head (or above the head of another person), from which the universal life energy of Reiki is bubbling.

Reiki Symbol

This is the term for the two Japanese characters, also called *Kanjis* that represent the Japanese expression "Reiki." In the more precise meaning of the word, this is actually not a symbol but simply the two Japanese characters that stand for "Rei" and "Ki." / *cf.: Ki, Rei, Symbols*

Reiki Teacher

In some styles of the Usui System, the term "Reiki Teacher" describes someone who has been initiated into the Third Degree and holds Reiki seminars. In other styles of the Usui System in which the Third Degree is divided into two levels, the term "Reiki Teacher" describes someone who has been initiated into the second level of the Third Degree, which is frequently called "3B," and is therefore entitled to hold Reiki seminars. In these styles, those who have just attained the first level of the Third Degree, meaning the initiation into the Third Degree, frequently called "3A," are given the name of "Reiki Master" but are not entitled to also teach the Usui System. In other styles of the Usui System, the term "Reiki Teacher" is not used at all. Because of the currently widespread subdivision of the Third Degree into the Master Degree and the Teacher Degree, we can observe that practitioners of the Third Degree in those styles that simply call themselves "Reiki Masters" (even though they also teach the Usui System) are now using the term "Reiki Master/Teacher" to avoid being possibly underrated and make it clear that they have not only received the initiation into the Third Degree but also teach the Usui System. / *cf.: Third Degree, Reiki Master, Reiki Master/Teacher*

Second Degree

The Second Degree of the Usui System of Reiki is generally taught within the framework of a three-day seminar. It is intended as an intensification of the personal path with Reiki and should not be taken until at least six months after the First Degree; however, a waiting period of at least one year or more is recommended in most cases. The seminar generally includes one initiation (in some styles of the Usui System there are also two or three), as well as learning the three related symbols. The participants practice the use of the symbols, which gives them the ability to intensify the flow of Reiki and to do the mental treatment and the distant treatment. / cf.: Initiation, First Degree, Third Degree

Second Symbol

See: Mental-Healing Symbol

Self-Treatment

This is a form of the treatment with Reiki in which the practitioners treat themselves. In many forms and further developments of the Usui System, self-treatment is considered to be the main component of the daily practice of the systems. / cf.: Individual Treatment, Group Treatment

Sensei

This expression is used by the Japanese to show respect for another person. For example, "Sensei" is added after the name of the person when someone speaks or writes about him or her. The use of the expression "Usui Sensei" for Mikao Usui is customary among Japanese Reiki practitioners. Furthermore, "Sensei" is also used in a general sense. In Japan, all teachers, professors, doctors, representatives, attorneys, and authors are called "Sensei."

Shinpiden

This is the Japanese word for the Third Reiki Degree and/or the Master Degree. "Shinpiden" means something like "teaching of the mysteries." / *cf.: Okuden, Shoden* / See pg. 30, pg. 42.

Shoden

This is the Japanese word for the First Reiki Degree. "Shoden" means something like "the fundamental teaching." / *cf.: Okuden, Shinpiden* / See pg. 30, pg. 44 ff.

Spiritual Lineage

There are nine elements within the *Usui Shiki Ryoho* that describe the form of the system (see pg. 93). The Spiritual Lineage is one of these nine elements. This does not mean the lineage or initiation lineage to which a person belongs who practices Reiki or teaches it but the lineage in which the respective Lineage Bearer of the *Usui Shiki Ryoho* stands. The role of the Lineage Bearer, also called Grand Master, is to watch over the integrity of the system in its essence and form. The Spiritual Lineage within the *Usui Shiki Ryoho* is currently the following: Mikao Usui—Dr. Chujiro Hayashi—Hawayo Takata—Phyllis Lei Furumoto. / *cf.: Grand Master, Lineage, Usui Shiki Ryoho* / See pg. 92 ff.

Students

In the Usui System of Reiki, this is the short form of the name for "Reiki students." Practitioners of the First and Second Degree are generally called "students," while those initiated into the Third Degree are called "Master," "Teacher," or "Master/Teacher." It is also obvious that the "Masters" or "Teachers" are aware that they will always remain "students of the universal life energy Reiki." / *cf.: Third Degree*

Symbols

On the one hand, a symbol is a sign; on the other hand, it is simultaneously much more than that: While a simple sign, such as a traffic sign, solely has an established, understandable significance, a symbol also contains the intimation of a deeper meaning. Here is an example: In the botanical garden, on the door of a greenhouse, there is a picture of a rose—a simple sign that there are roses in this greenhouse. However, if this same illustration of a rose is on a greeting card, for example, that is intended to send a greeting of love, then the rose is a symbol of deep love. The word symbol comes from the Greek word *Symballein,* which means something like "thrown or brought together." In ancient Greece, a *Symbolon* was a sign of recognition agreed to between friends consisting of two fragments (of a ring, for example), which resulted in a whole when "brought together." / *cf.: Distant-Healing Symbol, Power Symbol, Master Symbol, Mental-Healing Symbol, Reiki Symbol*

Teacher

This is used as the short form of "Reiki Teacher" in the Usui System of Reiki. / *cf.: Third Degree, Reiki Teacher, Reiki Master, Reiki Master/Teacher*

Teacher Degree

This term describes the Third Degree and sometimes the second level of the Third Degree. / *cf.: Third Degree, Master Degree, Reiki Teacher*

Teacher Training

See: Master Training

The Radiance Technique®

This technique is based on the Usui System of Reiki with a total of seven degrees, shaped by Dr. Barbara Ray. Dr. Barbara Ray is one of the 22 Masters who learned the Usui System of Reiki from Mrs. Takata. / See pg. 96.

The Reiki Alliance

This is an international association of Reiki Masters who practice the *Usui Shiki Ryoho* System in the tradition of Hawayo Takata. The Reiki Alliance was founded in 1982 in the USA and currently has about 600 members. The members acknowledge Phyllis Furumoto as the Lineage Bearer or Grand Master of the *Usui Shiki Ryoho*. / *cf.: Spiritual Lineage, Usui Shiki Ryoho*

The Reiki Association

Based in Great Britain, this is an organization for Reiki Masters and students that is open to English-speaking practitioners of the Usui System throughout the world. The Reiki Association, abbreviated as TRA, was founded in 1991 in Great Britain and currently has more than one-thousand members. The TRA is oriented upon the standards for the practice of the system issued by the Office of the Grand Master of the *Usui Reiki Ryoho* (see pg. 92 ff.) but is also open to practitioners from all directions of the Usui System.

The Reiki Network

This is an international association of Reiki Masters that was founded in 1990 by John and Esther Veltheim. Above all, the objectives of the association are networking, as well as the creation of mandatory teaching standards for all members. The Reiki Network currently has about 100 members. There are subordinate regional associations in various countries.

Third Degree

This is a term used for the Master Degree, which is sometimes also called the Teacher Degree or the Master/Teacher Degree. With the Third Degree, the students enter into a special connection with the initiating Master/Teacher. According to the style, the training to become a Master and/or teacher may last anywhere from several months to a number of years. Students should wait at least two to three years after receiving the First Degree to begin with the training. The Third Degree enables the initiated person to initiate others into the First, Second, and, if appropriate, the Third Degree. It is usually expected that a newly initiated Master/Teacher will only begin training other Masters/Teachers after a corresponding waiting period of several years; this is necessary for the individual to have sufficient experiences in the activities of a Master/Teacher, such as holding First Degree and Second Degree seminars. While some people who hold Reiki seminars call themselves "Reiki Masters," others use the words "Reiki Teacher." The term "Reiki Master/Teacher" is also widespread since both words are included here. The confusion of terms exists because the same terms sometimes have a different meaning in various forms of the Usui System: For example, while someone who is initiated into the Third Degree in *Usui Shiki Ryoho* is called a Master, which also means that he or she is simultaneously a teacher, there are other directions in which the Third Degree is divided into two levels, the Master Degree and the Teacher Degree. In this case, the Master Degree is frequently called "3A" and the Teacher Degree is "3B." Anyone who received the Master Degree, meaning the "3A" according to this system has obtained the initiation into the Third Degree but does not yet have the right to teach the Usui System; this only comes with the attainment of the Teacher Degree, "3B." In addition, there are forms of the Usui System in which the term "master" is dispensed with completely and only the word "teacher" is used. The different terms are related to the self-image of the respective person who is initiated into the Third Degree and/or the self-image predominating within the respective form of the Usui System in relation to the Third Degree. / *cf.: First Degree, Master Training, Reiki Teacher, Reiki Master, Reiki Master/Teacher, Second Degree.*

Third Symbol
See: Distant-Healing Symbol

Trademarks
See: Licensing

Treatment
When they give Reiki, some practitioners speak of a "Reiki treatment," but others use the term "Reiki application." The various terms are accompanied by different opinions as to the basic nature of giving Reiki. However, the use of specific terms may also have legal grounds.

Treatment of Other People
see: Individual Treatment

TRTIA
Abb. for: The Radiance Technique International Association. The current name of the organization founded in the late 1970s by Dr. Barbara Ray, one of the Masters initiated by Hawayo Takata, under the name of ARA (American Reiki Association). / *cf.: The Radiance Technique®*

Universal Life Energy
This is the general, customary translation for the Japanese term "Reiki." / *cf.: Ki, Rei, Reiki*

Usui Reiki Ryoho Gakkai
This phrase can be translated as the "Society for the Reiki Healing Method of Usui." The society was reportedly founded personally by Mikao Usui during his lifetime. Since the 1920s it has cultivated and preserved the Reiki healing method of Mikao Usui in its original form in Japan. / See pg. 37.

Usui Reiki Ryoho International (URRI)

This is an international network of Reiki Masters who share a special interest in "Japanese Reiki" with each other. After a workshop for "Japanese Reiki" was organized in August 1999 in Vancouver, Canada by six Reiki Masters from the USA, England, Canada, and Japan, in which about 70 Reiki Masters participated, some of them founded the *Usui Reiki Ryoho International*. This created a network in which a mutual exchange takes place, primarily through the Internet. During the four years after 1999, an additional workshop was organized every year: 2000 in Kyoto (Japan), 2001 in Madrid (Spain), 2002 in Toronto (Canada), and 2003 in Denmark.

Usui Shiki Ryoho

This can be translated as the "Usui System (or Method) of Healing," which is the current term for the system of Reiki that came to the Western world in 1938 via Hawaii. It was taught on Hawaii for the first time by Dr. Hayashi, together with Hawayo Takata. Shortly thereafter, he authorized her to also teach this practice. In the certificate signed by a notary public that Dr. Hayashi had prepared for Hawayo Takata, the practice was described in several different ways: "The Usui System of Reiki Healing," ,"The Usui Reiki System of Drugless Healing," and "Dr. Usui's Reiki System of Healing." Through Hawayo Takata, this system of Reiki reached mainland USA, from where it spread throughout the world at the beginning of the 1980s. / *cf.: Spiritual Lineage, The Reiki Alliance* / See pg. 92 ff.

Index of the Exercises/Texts by the Contributing Authors

Copyright Information

Exercises/Texts of the Contributing Authors:

Exercise "Hatsureiho Meditation" (pg. 22) was published with the friendly permission of Don Alexander.

Exercises "Reiki with a Bach Flower Essence" (pg. 186) and "Reiki with an Aura-Soma Essence" (pg. 194) were published with friendly permission of Anita Bind-Klinger.

Text "Contact to the Spiritual Guides" (pg. 226) was published with the friendly permission of Sabine Fennell.

Exercise "Reiki, Sound, and Gratitude" (pg. 215) was published with the friendly permission of Dagmar Fröhlich.

Text "The Way with Reiki" (pg. 147) was published with the friendly permission of Phyllis Lei Furumoto.

Exercise "Feeling the Heart Space" (pg. 125) was published with the friendly permission of Himani H. Gerber.

Exercise "Connecting with the Inner Peace" (pg. 182) was published with the friendly permission of Tanmaya Honervogt and Innenwelt Verlag, Cologne, Germany.

Exercise "The Energy of Breath" (pg. 242) was published with the friendly permission of Swami Prem Jagran.

Exercise "Cleansing the Spinal Column through Breathing" (pg. 170) was published with the friendly permission of Hiroko Kasahara.

Exercise "Reiki Treatment with Quartz Crystal" (pg. 200) was published with the friendly permission of Ursula Klinger-Omenka.

Exercise "Chakra Development with the Reiki Powerball" (pg. 108) was published with the friendly permission of Walter Lübeck.

Exercise "Process Oriented Movement Meditation" (pg. 248) was published with the friendly permission of Peter Mascher.

Text "Hawayo Takata's Directives" (pg. 78) and Exercise "Exploring my Anger" (pg. 89) were published with the friendly permission of Paul Mitchell.

Exercises "Byosen Partner Exercise" (pg. 48) and "Gassho Meditation" (pg. 152) were published with the friendly permission of Frank Arjava Petter.

Exercise "Harmonious Inner Communication" (pg. 132) was published with the friendly permission of Dr. Ranga Premaratna.

Text "Preparing for a Reiki Attunement" (pg. 140) was published with the friendly permission of William Lee Rand.

Exercise "Bipolar Energy Flow" (pg. 116) was published with the friendly permission of Edwin Zimmerli.

Longer Quotes or a Larger Number from One Work:

Quotes from the book *Reiki—Hawayo Takata' Story* (see chapter 2 and 3): Reprinted with permission from *Reiki—Hawayo Takata's Story* by Helen J. Haberly, pulished by Archedigm Publications, P. O. Box 1109, Olney, MD 20830. ©2000 All Rights Reserved.

Registered Trademarks:

Notes

Chapter 1: The Beginnings

1   A translation of the inscription is found in *Reiki Fire*, Frank Arjava Petter, Lotus Press, Twin Lakes/WI, 2001, pg. 28f.

2   From a German-language article about the inscription on the memorial stone of Mikao Usui (translated from Japanese by Hiroko Kasahara), *Reiki Magazin*, Issue 2/2003, pg. 38.

3   Ibid., pg. 40 / At the end of the inscription, Masayuki Okada, Ph.D. in Literature, was cited as the writer of the text. According to information from Hiroshi Doi, which I received through Hiroko Kasahara, Masayuki Okada was probably neither a member of the *Usui Reiki Ryoho Gakkai* nor initiated into Reiki. He was apparently commissioned to write the memorial-stone inscription because he was a well-known literary scholar and expert in the field of creating such inscriptions.

4   From a German-language article on Reiki in Japan by Hiroko Kasahara, *Reiki Magazin*, Issue 4/2003, pg. 39.

5   From a German-language article about the inscription on the memorial stone of Mikao Usui (translated from Japanese by Hiroko Kasahara), *Reiki Magazin*, Issue 2/2003, pg. 40.

6   Ibid., pg. 39.

7   From a booklet by Frank Arjava Petter for the CD *Reiki—Space of Peace and Love*, Merlin's Magic, translated by Christine M. Grimm, Inner Worlds Music, Twin Lakes/WI.

8   From a German-language article about the inscription on the memorial stone of Mikao Usui (translated from Japanese by Hiroko Kasahara), *Reiki Magazin*, Issue 2/2003, pg. 39.

9   All information in this paragraph comes from the German-language article on Reiki in Japan by Hiroko Kasahara, *Reiki Magazin*, Issue 4/2003, pg. 38f.

10 Ibid. / "Biography" means that he was familiar with the lives of famous people. "Shinsen" probably refers to the area of Shinsenism. This term describes the mysticism of ancient China, which was also integrated into Taoism. In addition, this term is also used synonymously for Taoism in Japanese. "Incantation" means the magical use of sounds, mantras, and songs. "Physiognomy" refers to the relationship between the shape of the human body and the character of an individual, as well as the associated ability to infer the inner characteristics on the basis of the physiognomy.

11 From an interview with Paul Mitchell about *Usui Shiki Ryoho*, Part 1, Oliver Klatt, published in German language in *Reiki Magazin*, Issue 2/2004, pg. 38 / For the interview in English language see the website: www.reiki-magazin.de, keyword "International", scroll down to: "Usui Shiki Ryoho"—an interview with Paul David Mitchell, October 2003.

12 From a German-language article about the inscription on the memorial stone of Mikao Usui (translated from Japanese by Hiroko Kasahara), *Reiki Magazin*, Issue 2/2003, pg. 38 / (*Gyo* = 1. light of dawn 2. clear, bright, 3. to be well-versed in something, to be familiar with something; *han* = sail)

13 Ibid., pg. 38f.

14 Ibid., pg. 39.

15 Ibid.

16 Ibid. / Hiroshi Doi writes: "In September 1923 the Great Kanto Earthquake occurred. It was a great disaster, 104,000 people killed or missing and 460,000 homes collapsed or destroyed by fire. Usui Sensei and his disciples roved the town the days following the quake, treating the wounded and saving innumerable people from death." (From "An Interview with Hiroshi Doi," William Lee Rand, *Reiki News Magazine*, Vol. Two, Issue Two, pg. 11.)

17 Ibid.

18 From a German-language article on Reiki in Japan by Hiroko Kasahara, *Reiki Magazin*, Issue 4/2003, pg. 38f.

19 *The Hayashi Reiki Manual* by Frank Arjava Petter, Tadao Yamaguchi, and Chujiro Hayashi, Lotus Press, Twin Lakes/WI, 2003, pg. 17.

20 From a German-language article on Reiki in Japan by Hiroko Kasahara, *Reiki Magazin*, Issue 4/2003, pg. 38.

21 Ibid., pg. 39.

22 *The Spirit of Reiki* by Walter Lübeck, Frank Arjava Petter, and William Lee Rand (translated by Christine M. Grimm), Lotus Press, Twin Lakes/WI, 2002, pg. 287.

23 From a German-language article on Reiki in Japan by Hiroko Kasahara, *Reiki Magazin*, Issue 4/2003, pg. 41.

24 At least this is what is written in the memorial-stone inscription (see German-language article about the inscription on the memorial stone of Mikao Usui, translated from Japanese by Hiroko Kasahara, *Reiki Magazin*, Issue 2/2003, pg. 39). According to another version, he died as a result of a stroke that he supposedly suffered while teaching a Reiki class. See *The Spirit of Reiki* by Walter Lübeck, Frank Arjava Petter, and William Lee Rand (translated by Christine M. Grimm), Lotus Press, Twin Lakes/WI, 2002, pg. 16.

25 *The Spirit of Reiki* by Walter Lübeck, Frank Arjava Petter, and William Lee Rand (translated by Christine M. Grimm), Lotus Press, Twin Lakes/WI, 2002, pg. 293.

Chapter 2: Continuation

1 From a German-language article about the inscription on the memorial stone of Mikao Usui (translated from Japanese by Hiroko Kasahara), *Reiki Magazin*, Issue 2/2003, pg. 40.

2 According to the research of Frank Arjava Petter and Dave King, there were 16 people (see *The Spirit of Reiki* by Walter Lübeck, Frank Arjava Petter, and William Lee Rand, Lotus Press, Twin Lakes/WI, 2002, pg. 17). According to the research by Hiroko Kasahara, there were 21 people, of whom eleven have been identified to date; among these eleven there were supposedly three women (see German-language article on Reiki in Japan by Hiroko Kasahara, *Reiki Magazin*, Issue 4/2003, pg. 40). A photo belonging to Tadao Yamaguchi shows Mikao Usui together with 20 men, all of whom were initiated by Usui into the Third Degree (*Shinpiden*).

3   *The Spirit of Reiki* by Walter Lübeck, Frank Arjava Petter, and William Lee Rand, Lotus Press, Twin Lakes/WI, 2002, pg. 17.

4   From a German-language article about Reiki in Japan by Hiroko Kasahara, *Reiki Magazin*, Issue 4/2003, pg. 40.

5   *The Spirit of Reiki* by Walter Lübeck, Frank Arjava Petter, and William Lee Rand, Lotus Press, Twin Lakes/WI, 2002, pg. 17.

6   From a German-language article about the inscription on the memorial stone of Mikao Usui (translated from Japanese by Hiroko Kasahara), *Reiki Magazin*, Issue 2/2003, pg. 40.

7   *Reiki—The Legacy of Dr. Usui* by Frank Arjava Petter (translated by Christine M. Grimm), Lotus Press, Twin Lakes/WI, 1998, pg. 13f.

8   Ibid. / According to Frank Arjava Petter, the phrase "security in life" should be understood as "securing one's own financial future." The term "descendents" means not only one's own family but also one's own students.

9   From a German-language article about Reiki in Japan by Hiroko Kasahara, *Reiki Magazin*, Issue 4/2003, pg. 41ff.

10   *Reiki Fire*, Frank Arjava Petter, Lotus Press, Twin Lakes/WI, 2001, pg. 21.

11   *The Hayashi Reiki Manual* by Frank Arjava Petter, Tadao Yamaguchi, and Chujiro Hayashi, Lotus Press, Twin Lakes/WI, 2003, pg. 13f. and a German-language article on Reiki in Japan by Hiroko Kasahara, *Reiki Magazin*, Issue 4/2003, pg. 40.

12   The rank of an admiral in the navy corresponds with that of a general in the army. So someone who has the rank of a general and is in the navy is called an admiral.

13   *The Hayashi Reiki Manual* by Frank Arjava Petter, Tadao Yamaguchi, and Chujiro Hayashi, Lotus Press, Twin Lakes/WI, 2003, pg. 13.

14   Ibid. / This also states that the 1935 address of the Hayashi family, out of which Dr. Hayashi also operated the Reiki clinic was the following: 28 Higashi-shinano-cho, Yotsuya, Tokyo (today: 27 Shinano-cho, Shinjuku ward, Tokyo).

15   From a German-language article on Reiki in Japan by Hiroko Kasahara, *Reiki Magazin*, Issue 4/2003, pg. 40.

16   *The Hayashi Reiki Manual* by Frank Arjava Petter, Tadao Yamaguchi, and Chujiro Hayashi, Lotus Press, Twin Lakes/WI, 2003, pg. 34.

17   Ibid., pg. 15f.

18   Ibid.

19   Ibid.

20   Ibid.

21   *Reiki: Hawayo Takata's Story* by Helen J. Haberly, Archedigm Publications, Olney/MD, 2000, and *Living Reiki: Takata's Teachings* by Fran Brown, LifeRhythm, Mendocino/CA, 1992.

22   *The Hayashi Reiki Manual* by Frank Arjava Petter, Tadao Yamaguchi, and Chujiro Hayashi, Lotus Press, Twin Lakes/WI, 2003, pg. 18f.

23   From a German-language article about Reiki in Japan by Hiroko Kasahara, *Reiki Magazin*, Issue 4/2003, pg. 38.

24   Ibid.

25   Ibid.

26 Ibid.

27 *The Hayashi Reiki Manual* by Frank Arjava Petter, Tadao Yamaguchi, and Chujiro Hayashi, Lotus Press, Twin Lakes/WI, 2003

28 Ibid., pg. 39f / a few changes have been made in the order of the exercise, with the friendly permission of Frank Arjava Petter.

29 *The Spirit of Reiki* by Walter Lübeck, Frank Arjava Petter, and William Lee Rand, Lotus Press, Twin Lakes/WI, 2002, pg. 36.

30 From a German-language article about Reiki in Japan by Hiroko Kasahara, *Reiki Magazin*, Issue 4/2003, pg. 40.

31 *The Hayashi Reiki Manual* by Frank Arjava Petter, Tadao Yamaguchi, and Chujiro Hayashi, Lotus Press, Twin Lakes/WI, 2003, pg. 16.

32 Ibid., pg. 33.

33 *Reiki: Hawayo Takata's Story* by Helen J. Haberly, Archedigm Publications, Olney/MD, 2000, pg. 17-19.

34 Ibid., pg. 17f.

35 Ibid., pg. 25-26.

36 Ibid., pg. 33.

37 Ibid.

38 *The Hayashi Reiki Manual* by Frank Arjava Petter, Tadao Yamaguchi, and Chujiro Hayashi, Lotus Press, Twin Lakes/WI, 2003, pg. 26.

39 Ibid., pg. 35 and a German-language article about Reiki in Japan by Hiroko Kasahara, *Reiki Magazin*, Issue 4/2003, pg. 40.

40 From a German-language article about Reiki in Japan by Hiroko Kasahara, *Reiki Magazin*, Issue 4/2003, pg. 40 and the copy of the certificate that Dr. Hayashi gave to Mrs. Takata in 1938 on Hawaii in *The Spirit of Reiki* by Walter Lübeck, Frank Arjava Petter, and William Lee Rand, Lotus Press, Twin Lakes/WI, 2002, pg. 301.

41 *The Hayashi Reiki Manual* by Frank Arjava Petter, Tadao Yamaguchi, and Chujiro Hayashi, Lotus Press, Twin Lakes/WI, 2003, pg. 27.

42 From a German-language article about Reiki in Japan by Hiroko Kasahara, *Reiki Magazin*, Issue 4/2003, pg. 40.

43 Ibid., pg. 38.

Chapter 3: Bridges into the West

1 From an interview with Paul Mitchell about *Usui Shiki Ryoho*, Part 1, Oliver Klatt, published in German language in *Reiki Magazin*, Issue 2/2004, pg. 39 / For the interview in English language see the website: www.reiki-magazin.de, keyword "International", scroll down to: "Usui Shiki Ryoho"—an interview with Paul David Mitchell, October 2003.

2 From an article about *Reiki Jin-Kei-Do*—The Path of Compassion and Wisdom through Reiki by Gordon Bell, published in German language in *Reiki Magazin*, Issue 2/2002, pg. 20f / For the article in English language see the website: www.reiki-magazin.de, keyword "International", scroll down to: "*Reiki Jin-Kei-Do*—The Path of Compassion and Wisdom through Reiki" by Gordon Bell.

3 *Living Reiki: Takata's Teachings* by Fran Brown, LifeRhythm, Mendocino/CA, 1992, pg. 14.

4   Ibid., pg. 16.

5   Ibid., pg. 18.

6   Ibid. / According to Phyllis Furumoto, her grandmother's maiden name was "Kawamura" and not "Kawamuru," as stated in the book by Fran Brown; this spelling has been corrected in the quote.

7   Ibid., pg. 25f.

8   *In the Light of a Distant Star* by Wanja Twan, Morning Star Productions, Vancouver, Canada, 1995, pg. 30-32 / Published with the friendly permission of Wanja Twan.

9   *Reiki: Hawayo Takata's Story* by Helen J. Haberly, Archedigm Publications, Olney/MD, 2000, pg. 27-28.

10 *Living Reiki: Takata's Teachings* by Fran Brown, LifeRhythm, Mendocino/CA, 1992, pg. 57.

11 *Reiki: Hawayo Takata's Story* by Helen J. Haberly, Archedigm Publications, Olney/MD, 2000, pg. 33.

12 Ibid., pg. 33f. and *The Spirit of Reiki* by Walter Lübeck, Frank Arjava Petter, and William Lee Rand, Lotus Press, Twin Lakes/WI, 2002, pg. 301.

13 *The Spirit of Reiki* by Walter Lübeck, Frank Arjava Petter, and William Lee Rand, Lotus Press, Twin Lakes/WI, 2002, pg. 301 and an interview with Paul Mitchell about *Usui Shiki Ryoho*, Part 1, Oliver Klatt, published in German language in *Reiki Magazin*, Issue 2/2004, pg. 38 / For the interview in English language see the website: www.reiki-magazin.de, keyword "International", scroll down to: "*Usui Shiki Ryoho*"—an interview with Paul David Mitchell, October 2003.

14 All of the information from this paragraph and the following one come from *Reiki: Hawayo Takata's Story* by Helen J. Haberly, Archedigm Publications, Olney/MD, 2000, pg. 35f.

15 Ibid., pg. 43-44.

16 *Living Reiki: Takata's Teachings* by Fran Brown, LifeRhythm, Mendocino/CA, 1992, and *Reiki: Hawayo Takata's Story* by Helen J. Haberly, Archedigm Publications, Olney/MD, 2000.

17 First section quoted from "First Person: Mrs. Takata Tells Her Story. A Daughter's Remorse. The Mother's Funeral: Part 1," *Reiki Magazine International*, Issue 7 (Oct./Nov. 2000), pg. 33 / Second section, starting at "Suddenly she looked at me" quoted from "What is Reiki? Cancel the Funeral. The Mother's Funeral. Part 2," *Reiki Magazine International*, Issue 8 (Dec. 2000/Jan. 2001), pg. 9 / Both excerpts are transcriptions from a tape recording —publication in *Reiki Magazine International* with the permission of John Harvey Gray and Lourdes Gray, who own the tape recording.

18 *Reiki: Hawayo Takata's Story* by Helen J. Haberly, Archedigm Publications, Olney/MD, 2000, pg. 45-46.

19 "Interview with Reiki Masters Initiated by Hawayo Takata—Barbara Brown" by Rolf Holm, *Reiki Magazine International*, Issue 1 (Oct./Nov. 1999), pg. 27.

20 "We Are All Healers," *Reiki Magazine International*, Issue 1 (Oct./Nov. 1999), pg. 8 / is excerpted from the paperback by Sally Hammond about Hawayo Takata, published in 1973 by Ballantine Books with the title *We are All Healers*.

21 "Fifty Years of Reiki: Toshiko Takaezo Remembers Takata" by Bill Stucky, *Reiki Magazine International*, Issue 7 (Oct./Nov. 2000), pg. 25.

22 *Living Reiki: Takata's Teachings* by Fran Brown, LifeRhythm, Mendocino/CA, 1992, pg. 92.

23 From a brochure that was compiled by Alice Takata Furumoto, the daughter of Hawayo Takata and mother of Phyllis Furumoto, in 1982 and given to Masters initiated by Takata (also known as *The Gray Book* under the title of *"Leiki"* / cf. Chapter 4).

24 cf. Chapter 1

25 "In Context: Applying the Reiki Precepts to the Practice. A Conversation with Phyllis Furumoto" by Barbara McDaniel, *Reiki Magazine International*, Issue 18 (August/September 2002), pg. 7.

26 *Reiki: Hawayo Takata's Story* by Helen J. Haberly, Archedigm Publications, Olney/MD, 2000, pg. 50-51.

27 *The Original Reiki Handbook of Dr. Mikao Usui*, edited by Frank Arjava Petter, Lotus Press, Twin Lakes/WI, 2000, pg. 27f. and *The Hayashi Reiki Manual* by Frank Arjava Petter, Tadao Yamaguchi, and Chujiro Hayashi, Lotus Press, Twin Lakes/WI, 2003, pg. 63f. / However, it appears that Mikao Usui also did not rule out any form of self-treatment. In the second section of the *Reiki Ryoho Hikkei*, the "Handbook of the Reiki Method of Healing" (cf. Chapter 6), which consists of questions (from Usui's students) and answers (from Usui) we read the following: "Question: With it (the *Usui Reiki Ryoho*), other people can be healed. But what about oneself? Can a person also heal his own health disorders? Answer: If we cannot heal our own diseases, then how should we heal others?" from: *Reiki—The Legacy of Dr. Usui* by Frank Arjava Petter (translated by Christine M. Grimm), Lotus Press, Twin Lakes/WI, 1998, pg. 19.

28 *The Original Reiki Handbook of Dr. Mikao Usui*, edited by Frank Arjava Petter, Lotus Press, Twin Lakes/WI, 2000, pg. 31.

29 *The Hayashi Reiki Manual* by Frank Arjava Petter, Tadao Yamaguchi, and Chujiro Hayashi, Lotus Press, Twin Lakes/WI, 2003, pg. 64.

30 *The Reiki Sourcebook* by Bronwen and Frans Stiene, O Books, Winchester/UK, New York/USA, 2003, pg. 78f.

31 Ibid. pg. 81.

32 Ibid. pg. 153.

33 "We Are All Healers," *Reiki Magazine International*, Issue 1 (Oct./Nov. 1999) / is excerpted from the paperback by Sally Hammond about Hawayo Takata, published in 1973 by Ballantine Books with the title *We are All Healers*.

34 *Die Heilkraft des Reiki. Lehren einer Meisterin* by Mary McFadyen (German-language book), Rowohlt Taschenbuch Verlag, Hamburg, 2000, pg. 16, and *The Reiki Sourcebook* by Bronwen and Frans Stiene, O Books, Winchester/UK, New York/USA, 2003, pg. 149 (cited as a source: *Hand to Hand* by John Harvey Gray, Xlibris Corporation, 2002).

35 *Living Reiki: Takata's Teachings* by Fran Brown, LifeRhythm, Mendocino/CA, 1992, pg. 60.

36 "Mrs. Takata's Masters. A series of conversations with Reiki Masters initiated by Hawayo Takata. John Gray" by Rolf Holm, *Reiki Magazine International*, Issue 7 (Oct./Nov. 2000), pg. 18.

37 *The Reiki Sourcebook* by Bronwen and Frans Stiene, O Books, Winchester/UK, New York/USA, 2003, pg. 151.

38 "Phyllis Lei Furumoto. Choosing Reiki. My Reiki Story—Part I" by Phyllis Furumoto, edited by Barbara McDaniel, *Reiki Magazine International*, Issue 7 (Oct./Nov. 2000), pg. 7.

39 Ibid., pg. 5f.

40 Ibid., pg. 9.

41 *Die Radiance Technik* by Ulrike Wolf (German-language book), Wilhelm Goldmann Verlag, München, 1999, pg. 236.

42 From the website: www.trtia.org, "Historical Perspectives on The Radiance Technique®, Authentic Reiki®, Real Reiki®, TRT®" by Dr. Barbara Ray / www.trtia.org/histpers.html (March 29, 2005).

43 Ibid.

44 "Mrs. Takata's Masters. A series of conversations with Reiki Masters initiated by Hawayo Takata. Paul Mitchell" by Rolf Holm, *Reiki Magazine International*, Issue 6 (Aug./Sept. 2000), pg. 19.

45 *Die Heilkraft des Reiki. Lehren einer Meisterin* by Mary McFadyen (German-language book), Rowohlt Taschenbuch Verlag, Hamburg, 2000, pg. 24f / Quote from the original English-language manuscript, which Mary McFadyen was kind enough to send me.

46 Ibid., pg. 25 / Quote from the original English-language manuscript, which Mary McFadyen was kind enough to send me.

47 Ibid., pg. 25f.

48 Ibid., pg. 25.

49 *The Reiki Sourcebook* by Bronwen and Frans Stiene, O Books, Winchester/UK, New York/USA, 2003, pg. 328.

50 Ibid., pg. 305.

51 "Interview with Reiki Masters Initiated by Hawayo Takata: Barbara Brown" by Rolf Holm, *Reiki Magazine International*, Issue 1 (Oct./Nov. 1999), pg. 27.

52 *Reiki: Hawayo Takata's Story* by Helen J. Haberly, Archedigm Publications, Olney/MD, 2000, pg. 47f.

53 Excerpt from a letter written by Mrs. Takata on January 17, 1980 in the *Reiki Magazine International*, Issue 6 (Aug./Sept. 2000), pg. 28.

54 *Reiki: Hawayo Takata's Story* by Helen J. Haberly, Archedigm Publications, Olney/MD, 2000, pg. 111.

55 *The Reiki Sourcebook* by Bronwen and Frans Stiene, O Books, Winchester/UK, New York/USA, 2003, pg. 159.

56 During a personal conversation in June 2004 in Cataldo, Idaho.

57 "Mrs. Takata Opens Minds to Reiki," *Reiki Magazine International*, Issue 2 (Dec. 1999/Jan. 2000), reprint from an article in the San Mateo Times (California) of May 17, 1975.

Chapter 4: Different Paths

1 *Die Heilkraft des Reiki. Lehren einer Meisterin* by Mary McFadyen (German-language book), Rowohlt Taschenbuch Verlag, Hamburg, 2000, pg. 16, and *The Reiki Sourcebook* by Bronwen and Frans Stiene, O Books, Winchester/UK, New York/USA, 2003, pg. 151f and *The Spirit of Reiki* by Walter Lübeck, Frank Arjava Petter, and William Lee Rand, Lotus Press, Twin Lakes/WI, 2002, pg. 19.

2   "Mrs. Takata's Masters. A series of conversations with Reiki Masters initiated by Hawayo Takata: John Gray," Rolf Holm, *Reiki Magazine International*, Issue 7 (Oct./Nov. 2000), pg. 18.

3   "The Work of a Lineage Bearer. My Reiki Story—Part 2" by Phyllis Furumoto with Barbara McDaniel, *Reiki Magazine International*, Issue 8 (Dec./Jan. 2001), pg. 4.

4   "Phyllis Lei Furumoto. Choosing Reiki. My Reiki Story—Part I" by Phyllis Furumoto, edited by Barbara McDaniel, *Reiki Magazine International*, Issue 7 (Oct./Nov. 2000), pg. 9.

5   *The Reiki Sourcebook* by Bronwen and Frans Stiene, O Books, Winchester/ UK, New York/USA, 2003, pg. 160 / Phyllis Furumoto told me in a personal conversation in June 2004 in Cataldo, Idaho that the meeting took place at the home of Barbara Brown.

6   *The Blue Book* by Paul David Mitchell and Phyllis Lei Furumoto, revised edition for The Reiki Alliance, Coeur d'Alene/ID, 1985 / This is a booklet that Reiki Masters who are members of The Reiki Alliance can order to give to their students in their own Reiki seminars, for example.

7   Ibid.

8   From the founding document of The Reiki Alliance / A copy of this document has been on the noticeboard at the conference of The Reiki Alliance in Gersfeld, Germany, in 2002.

9   "Mrs. Takata's Masters. A series of conversations with Reiki Masters initiated by Hawayo Takata. John Gray," Rolf Holm, *Reiki Magazine International*, Issue 7 (Oct./Nov. 2000), pg. 18 (on John Gray), as well as "Mrs. Takata's Masters. Interview with Reiki Masters initiated by Hawayo Takata. Fran Brown," Rolf Holm, *Reiki Magazine International*, Issue 5 (June/July 2000), pg. 18 (on Fran Brown) and *The Reiki Sourcebook* by Bronwen and Frans Stiene, O Books, Winchester/UK, New York/USA, 2003, pg. 162 (on Virginia Samdahl).

10 "The truth Is in Our Own Hands. An Interview with Phyllis Furumoto" by Oliver Klatt, *Reiki Magazine International*, Issue 15 (Feb./March 2002), pg. 7.

11 From an interview with Paul Mitchell on *Usui Shiki Ryoho*, Part I, by Oliver Klatt, published in German language in *Reiki Magazin*, Issue 2/2004, pg. 38 / For the interview in English language see the website: www.reiki-magazin.de, keyword "International", scroll down to: "Usui Shiki Ryoho"—an interview with Paul David Mitchell, October 2003.

12 *Die Heilkraft des Reiki. Lehren einer Meisterin* by Mary McFadyen (German-language book), Rowohlt Taschenbuch Verlag, Hamburg, 2000, pg. 17 / Quote from the original English-language manuscript, which Mary McFadyen was kind enough to send me.

13 *Die Radiance Technik* by Ulrike Wolf (German-language book), Wilhelm Goldmann Verlag, München, 1999, pg. 243.

14 "Mrs. Takata's Masters. Interview with Reiki Masters initiated by Hawayo Takata. Fran Brown," by Rolf Holm, *Reiki Magazine International*, Issue 5 (June/July 2000), pg. 18.

15 *The Reiki Sourcebook* by Bronwen and Frans Stiene, O Books, Winchester/ UK, New York/USA, 2003, pg. 328 / Paul Mitchell told me in a personal conversation, which took place in June 2004 in Cataldo, Idaho, that Dr. Barbara Ray was initiated by Virginia Samdahl into the 1st and 2nd Reiki Degree.

16 "Mrs. Takata's Masters. Interview with Reiki Masters initiated by Hawayo Takata. Fran Brown," Rolf Holm, *Reiki Magazine International,* Issue 5 (June/July 2000), pg. 18.

17 "The Work of a Lineage Bearer. My Reiki Story—Part 2" by Phyllis Furumoto, with Barbara McDaniel, *Reiki Magazine International,* Issue 8 (Dec./Jan. 2001), pg. 4.

18 Ibid.

19 This is the gist of what Phyllis Furumoto said at the Reiki Festival 2002 in Gersfeld, Germany, in October 2002.

20 *The Reiki Sourcebook* by Bronwen and Frans Stiene, O Books, Winchester/UK, New York/USA, 2003, pg. 311.

21 Ibid.

22 Ibid., pg. 319.

23 *Die Heilkraft des Reiki. Lehren einer Meisterin* by Mary McFadyen (German-language book), Rowohlt Taschenbuch Verlag, Hamburg, 2000, pg. 16f / Quote from the original English-language manuscript, which Mary McFadyen was kind enough to send me.

24 According to information from *The Reiki Sourcebook* (Glossary starting on pg. 303), from various articles in the *Reiki Magazine International,* and information from Barbara McDaniel and Phyllis Furumoto.

25 *The Reiki Sourcebook* by Bronwen and Frans Stiene, O Books, Winchester/UK, New York/USA, 2003, pg. 319f.

26 Ibid., pg. 319.

27 Ibid., pg. 327.

28 Ibid, pg. 163f.

29 Ibid, pg. 315f.

30 From an interview with Paul Mitchell on *Usui Shiki Ryoho,* Part 1, by Oliver Klatt, published in German language in *Reiki Magazin,* Issue 2/2004, pg. 40 / For the interview in English language see the website: www.reiki-magazin.de, keyword "International", scroll down to: "Usui Shiki Ryoho"—an interview with Paul David Mitchell, October 2003.

31 Ibid.

32 As Paul Mitchell describes it, he and Phyllis Furumoto had the opportunity to sit down together with George Araki, Wanja Twan, Fran Brown, John Gray, Beth Gray, Shinobu Saito, and Mary McFadyen. All of them agreed, as did he and Phyllis Furumoto, that the description of the system in the form of the four aspects and nine elements matched their perceptions of what they had received. In addition, Rick Bockner supposedly gave the same feedback.

33 "The Wheel of Reiki" by Phyllis Furumoto, Reiki Info (Swiss Reiki Magazine), Issue 1/1995, pg. 7f.

34 From an interview with Paul Mitchell on *Usui Shiki Ryoho,* Part 1, by Oliver Klatt, published in German language in *Reiki Magazin,* Issue 2/2004, pg. 38 / For the interview in English language see the website: www.reiki-magazin.de, keyword "International", scroll down to: "Usui Shiki Ryoho"—an interview with Paul David Mitchell, October 2003.

35 "Form and Freedom. An Interview with Paul Mitchell", Part 1, by Oliver Klatt, *Reiki Magazine International,* Issue 20 (Dec. 2002/January 2003), pg. 16.

36 From an interview with Paul Mitchell on *Usui Shiki Ryoho*, Part 1, by Oliver Klatt, published in German language in *Reiki Magazin*, Issue 2/2004, pg. 42 / For the interview in English language see the website: www.reiki-magazin.de, keyword "International", scroll down to: "Usui Shiki Ryoho"—an interview with Paul David Mitchell, October 2003.

37 Ibid., pg. 41.

38 *The Blue Book* by Paul David Mitchell and Phyllis Lei Furumoto, revised edition for The Reiki Alliance, Coeur d'Alene/ID, 1985 / This is a booklet that Reiki Masters who are members of The Reiki Alliance can order to give to their students in their own Reiki seminars, for example.

39 *The Reiki Factor. A Guide to Natural Healing, Helping, and Wholeness* by Barbara Weber Ray, Ph.D., Exposition Press, Smithtown/NY, 1983.

40 From the website: www.trtia.org, "Historical Perspectives on The Radiance Technique®, Authentic Reiki®, Real Reiki®, TRT®" by Dr. Barbara Ray / www.trtia.org/histpers.html (March 29, 2005).

41 Ibid.

42 Ibid.

43 Ibid.

44 From a German-language article on The Radiance Technique® by Frank Doerr, *Reiki Magazin*, Issue 4/2003, pg. 25.

45 The blurb on the cover of the first edition of *The Reiki Factor* says the following about Barbara Weber Ray, Ph.D.: "A Reiki Master, she received full training as a Third Degree Reiki Initiator in 1979." In Chapter 5 on "The Technique of Reiki" Barbara Weber Ray writes: "The Reiki method has been kept intact in its essence as it has been preserved and transmitted through the centuries. It is composed of three main levels or degrees." (page 27, 28) Furthermore, Dr. Ray writes: "An analogy to these three degrees of Reiki can be made to three degrees from a university. The First Degree of Reiki is analogous to the B.A., which gives the student a firm basis of knowledge that can be used with success throughout his or her life. The M.A. degree takes the student deeper into specific areas, and the Ph.D. is another dimension entirely beyond the previous two degrees. Similarly, the Second and Third degrees delve more deeply into the Reiki technique." (page 28) / *The Reiki Factor. A Guide to Natural Healing, Helping, and Wholeness* by Barbara Weber Ray, Ph.D., Exposition Press, Smithtown/NY, 1983.

46 *Die Radiance Technik* by Ulrike Wolf (German-language book), Luechow Verlag, Stuttgart, 2004, pg. 12 and pg. 22.

47 "Mrs. Takata's Masters. Interview with Reiki Masters Initiated by Hawayo Takata. Barbara Brown" by Rolf Holm, *Reiki Magazine International*, Issue 1, (Oct./Nov. 1999), pg. 25.

48 Ibid, pg. 26.

49 "Living with One Another" by Paul Mitchell, *Reiki Magazine International*, Issue 28, (April/May 2004), pg. 12.

50 Ibid., pg. 13.

Chapter 5: The Variety

1 From a German-language article on *Rainbow Reiki:* "Spiritual Energy Work and Personality Development for the Age of Aquarius" by Walter Lübeck, *Reiki Magazin* Special Edition in cooperation with the Windpferd publishing company, 2002, pg. 10.

2 Ibid.

3 From a German-language article on Walter Lübeck: A Portrait by Sylvia-Manuela Regler, *Reiki Magazin*, Issue 4/2002, pg. 48. Brigitte Müller received her Master initiation in 1983 from Phyllis Furumoto.

4 Ibid.

5 Ibid.

6 *Reiki—Best Practices* by Walter Lübeck and Frank Arjava Petter, translated by Christine M. Grimm, Lotus Press, Twin Lakes/WI, 2003, pg. 23f.

7 *Rainbow Reiki* by Walter Lübeck, translated by Christine M. Grimm, Lotus Press, Twin Lakes/WI, 1997, pg. 9.

8 From a German-language article on *Rainbow Reiki:* "Spiritual Energy Work and Personality Development for the Age of Aquarius" by Walter Lübeck, *Reiki Magazin* Special Edition in cooperation with the Windpferd publishing company, 2002, pg. 11.

9 Ibid.

10 Ibid, pg. 15.

11 Ibid., pg. 12.

12 Ibid., pg. 13.

13 Ibid.

14 Ibid., pg. 12.

15 Ibid., pg. 14.

16 *Rainbow Reiki*, pg. 30ff / A few changes have been made in the order of the exercise with the friendly permission of Walter Lübeck.

17 Ibid., pg. 29.

18 Ibid., pg. 15f.

19 From a German-language article on *Rainbow Reiki:* "Spiritual Energy Work and Personality Development for the Age of Aquarius" by Walter Lübeck, *Reiki Magazin* Special Edition in cooperation with the Windpferd Verlag publishing company, 2002, pg. 15.

20 From a German-language article on *Rei-Ki-Balancing®:* "The Reiki Power in the Earth Connection" by Gerda E. Drescher, *Reiki Magazin*, Issue 2/2003, pg. 22.

21 Ibid., pg. 22ff.

22 Ibid., pg. 24f / For reasons of clarity, this excerpt was changed in one place at the request of Edwin Zimmerli.

23 Ibid., pg. 25.

24 From written material on *Rei-Ki-Balancing®* that is partially unpublished, which Edwin Zimmerli was kind enough to send to me.

25 Ibid.

26 From a German-language article on *Rei-Ki-Balancing®:* "The Reiki Power in the Earth Connection" by Gerda E. Drescher, *Reiki Magazin*, Issue 2/2003, pg. 25.

27 According to Edwin Zimmerli this information comes from an excerpt of the book *What is LightBody?* by Tashira Tachi-ren

28 From written material on *Rei-Ki-Balancing®* that is partially unpublished, which Edwin Zimmerli was kind enough to send to me.

29 Ibid.

30 Ibid.

31 From a German-language article on *Osho Neo-Reiki* by Himani H. Gerber, *Reiki Magazin*, Issue 1/2003, pg. 42.

32 Ibid.

33 Ibid.

34 While Himani H. Gerber wrote about three initiations for the First Degree in the German-language article on *Osho Neo-Reiki* that appeared in the *Reiki Magazin*, Issue 1/2003, she later told me that she actually gives four initiations for the First Degree; she initially just spoke of three initiations because she combines two of the total of four initiations of the First Degree.

35 Ibid., pg. 43.

36 Ibid. / Also see the previously unpublished German-language manuscript about *Neo-Reiki:* "New Dimensions of Your Transformation and Creativity" by Himani H. Gerber, pg. 63f, which Himani was kind enough to send me.

37 From the previously unpublished German-language manuscript on *Neo-Reiki:* "New Dimensions of Your Transformation and Creativity" by Himani H. Gerber, Chapter 1: "Letting Go of the Old," pg. 8.

38 From a German-language article on *Osho Neo-Reiki* by Himani H. Gerber, *Reiki Magazin*, Issue 1/2003, pg. 42.

39 Ibid., pg. 43.

40 From the previously unpublished German-language manuscript about *Neo-Reiki:* "New Dimensions of Your Transformation and Creativity" by Himani H. Gerber, Chapter 4: "Sharing," pg. 71.

41 Ibid.

42 From a German-language article on *Osho Neo-Reiki* by Himani H. Gerber, *Reiki Magazin*, Issue 1/2003, pg. 43. At the request of Himani, the new term "metaphysical energy work" is used here instead of the old term "expanded energy work" that is used in the article.

43 Ibid.

44 From the previously unpublished German-language manuscript about *Neo-Reiki:* "New Dimensions of Your Transformation and Creativity" by Himani H. Gerber, Chapter 4: "Sharing," pg. 78.

45 Ibid.

46 Ibid., pg. 64f.

47 From an article about *Reiki Jin-Kei-Do:* "The Path of Compassion and Wisdom through Reiki" by Gordon Bell, published in German language in *Reiki Magazin*, Issue 2/2002, pg. 21 / For the article in English language see the website: www.reiki-magazin.de, keyword "International", scroll down to: *"Reiki Jin-Kei-Do:* The Path of Compassion and Wisdom through Reiki" by Gordon Bell.

48 Ibid.

49 Ibid., pg. 20f.

50 "Journey of a Reiki Lineage. Reiki Jin Kei Do" by Jim Frew, *Reiki Magazine International* (Issue 10, April/May 2001), pg. 19.

51 From the website by Gordon and Dorothy Bell: www.healing-touch.co.uk, "Introduction to EnerSense-Buddho," first sentence (May 2004).

52 Ibid., "History of Buddho-EnerSense" presents a summary.

53 "Journey of a Reiki Lineage. Reiki Jin Kei Do" by Jim Frew, *Reiki Magazine International* (Issue 10, April/May 2001), pg. 19.

54 From an article about *Reiki Jin-Kei-Do:* "The Path of Compassion and Wisdom through Reiki" by Gordon Bell, published in German language in *Reiki Magazin*, Issue 2/2002, pg. 21.

55 From the website by Gordon and Dorothy Bell: www.healing-touch.co.uk, "Letter from Ranga Premaratna regarding Kathleen Milner Comments," third paragraph (May 2004).

56 From an article about *Reiki Jin-Kei-Do:* "The Path of Compassion and Wisdom" through Reiki by Gordon Bell, published in German language in *Reiki Magazin*, Issue 2/2002, pg. 21.

57 "Journey of a Reiki Lineage. Reiki Jin Kei Do" by Jim Frew, *Reiki Magazine International* (Issue 10, April/May 2001), pg. 19.

58 From the website by Gordon and Dorothy Bell: www.healing-touch.co.uk, "Letter from Ranga Premaratna regarding Kathleen Milner Comments," fourth paragraph (May 2004).

59 "Journey of a Reiki Lineage. Reiki Jin Kei Do" by Jim Frew, *Reiki Magazine International* (Issue 10, April/May 2001), pg. 19.

60 From an article about *Reiki Jin-Kei-Do:* The Path of Compassion and Wisdom through Reiki by Gordon Bell, published in German language in *Reiki Magazin*, Issue 2/2002, pg. 21.

61 Ibid., pg. 22f.

62 Ibid., pg. 23.

63 Ibid.

64 Ibid.

65 According to Dr. Ranga Premaratna this exercise is one of the basic elements of *Reiki Jin Kei-Do.*

66 From an article about *Reiki Jin-Kei-Do:* "The Path of Compassion and Wisdom through Reiki" by Gordon Bell, published in German language in *Reiki Magazin*, Issue 2/2002, pg. 22.

67 Ibid.

68 From the website by Gordon and Dorothy Bell: www.healing-touch.co.uk, "Who can study Buddho-EnerSense" (May 2004).

69 "Journey of a Reiki Lineage. Reiki Jin Kei-Do" by Jim Frew, *Reiki Magazine International* (Issue 10, April/May 2001), pg. 19.

70 The information in this paragraph comes from the following books: *The Spirit of Reiki* by Walter Lübeck, Frank Arjava Petter, and William Lee Rand, Lotus Press, Twin Lakes/WI, 2002, pg. 297, and *Reiki: The Healing Touch* by William Lee Rand, Vision Publications, Southfield/MI, 2000, pg. iv.

71 From an article on Karuna Reiki® by William Lee Rand, published in German language in *Reiki Magazin*, Issue 4/2002, pg. 18 / for the article in English language see the website: www.reiki-magazin.de, keyword "International", scroll down to: "Karuna Reiki®" by William Lee Rand.

72 Ibid.

73 Ibid.

74 Ibid., pg. 19.

75 *The Book On Karuna Reiki®* by Laurelle Shanti Gaia, Infinite Light Healing Studies Center, Inc., Hartsel/CO, 2002, pg. 21.

76 Ibid., pg. 29.

77 Ibid., pg. 34.

78 Ibid., pg. 34 and pg. 109.

79 Ibid., pg. 34.

80 Ibid., pg. 27.

81 Ibid., pg. 142ff.

82 From an article on *Karuna Reiki®* by William Lee Rand, published in German language in *Reiki Magazin*, Issue 4/2002, pg. 18

83 Ibid.

84 Ibid.

85 Ibid., pg. 20.

86 Ibid.

87 *Reiki: The Healing Touch* by William Lee Rand, Vision Publications, Southfield/MI, 2000, pg. C-5f.

88 *The Reiki Sourcebook* by Bronwen and Frans Stiene, O Books, Winchester/UK, New York/USA, 2003, pg. 257f.

89 For example, there are numerous errors in the individual texts on the website of Kathleen Milner, the founder of *Tera-Mai Reiki* (www.kathleenmilner.com / May 2004), such as those in "What is Tera Mai?": The fifth paragraph states: "Takata founded the Alliance Reiki group and the initiations that were given were the Alliance Reiki attunements." There is neither an "Alliance Reiki group" (the correct name of the organization is "The Reiki Alliance") nor did Takata found The Reiki Alliance (it was established about two years after Takata's death / cf. Chap. 4). There are also no "Alliance Reiki attunements" (instead there is within the *Usui Shiki Ryoho* a certain form of doing initiations and the members of The Reiki Alliance understand themselves as Masters who practise and teach the *Usui Shiki Ryoho*; but this does not mean that all Masters who teach *Usui Shiki Ryoho* are members of The Reiki Alliance).

Chapter 6: The Rediscovery

1 *Reiki Fire*, Frank Arjava Petter, Lotus Press, Twin Lakes/WI, 2001, pg. 6.

2 *Reiki—The Legacy of Dr. Usui* by Frank Arjava Petter (translated by Christine M. Grimm), Lotus Press, Twin Lakes/WI, 1998, pg. 111.

3 Ibid., pg. 93f., as well as *Reiki Fire*, pg. 12f and the interview with Frank Arjava Petter (in French) "Sur les traces de Mikao Usui," Reiki Do Info (French Reiki Magazine), Numéro de lancement, Avril 2004, pg. 4-5.

4   *Reiki—The Legacy of Dr. Usui* by Frank Arjava Petter (translated by Christine M. Grimm), Lotus Press, Twin Lakes/WI, 1998, pg. 99f and *Reiki Fire*, Frank Arjava Petter, Lotus Press, Twin Lakes/WI, 2001, pg. 21.

5   *Reiki—The Legacy of Dr. Usui* by Frank Arjava Petter (translated by Christine M. Grimm), Lotus Press, Twin Lakes/WI, 1998, pg. 100f / As Frank Arjava Petter told me, this "Mrs. Koyama" was Kimiko Koyama, the President of the *Usui Reiki Ryoho Gakkai* at that time. Also see the interview with Frank Arjava Petter (in French) "Sur les traces de Mikao Usui," Reiki Do Info (French Reiki Magazine), Numéro de lancement, Avril 2004, pg. 4-5.

6   *Reiki—The Legacy of Dr. Usui* by Frank Arjava Petter (translated by Christine M. Grimm), Lotus Press, Twin Lakes/WI, 1998, pg. 109 / Also see the interview with Frank Arjava Petter (in French) "Sur les traces de Mikao Usui," Reiki Do Info (French Reiki Magazine), Numéro de lancement, Avril 2004, pg. 4-5: Frank Arjava Petter: "M. Oishi lui apportera lors d'une seconde séance de soins chez elle, la photo de Mikao Usui (le poster publié dans Feu de Reiki), que sa propre mère initiée au second degré, avait reçu en cadeau de son maitre Mikao Usui. Puis il révéla à Mme Akimoto, l'existence du 'Reiki Usui Ryoho Gakkai', et lui proposa de rencontrer l'un des dirigeants de la seconde branche de l'organisation, M. Ogawa, alors agé de plus de 90 ans. (…) …, j'ai demandé à mon élève de donner un traitement Reiki à M. Ogawa, qui fut ravi de sa séance. Il lui enseigna à son tour sa façon de faire 'à la japonaise' qui était différente. Shizuko m'a ensuite transmis l'enseignement de M. Ogawa, dont j'ai reçu plus tard le manuel de cours."

7   *Reiki—The Legacy of Dr. Usui* by Frank Arjava Petter (translated by Christine M. Grimm), Lotus Press, Twin Lakes/WI, 1998, pg. 27.

8   *Reiki Fire*, Frank Arjava Petter, Lotus Press, Twin Lakes/WI, 2001, pg. 25f.

9   *The Original Reiki Handbook of Dr. Mikao Usui*, edited by Frank Arjava Petter, Lotus Press, Twin Lakes/WI, 2000, pg. 15f / Reprint of the Gassho Meditation with the friendly permission of Frank Arjava Petter.

10 *The Reiki Sourcebook* by Bronwen and Frans Stiene, O Books, Winchester/UK, New York/USA, 2003, pg. 136.

11 *The Original Reiki Handbook of Dr. Mikao Usui*, edited by Frank Arjava Petter, Lotus Press, Twin Lakes/WI, 2000, pg. 7.

12 German-language interview with Frank A. Petter on Usui's Legacy by Oliver Klatt, *Reiki Magazin*, Issue 2/2000, pg. 11.

13 *The Reiki Sourcebook* by Bronwen and Frans Stiene, O Books, Winchester/UK, New York/USA, 2003, pg. 107.

14 Ibid., pg. 108

15 The complete text of the *Usui Reiki Ryoho Kyogi* is in *Reiki—The Legacy of Dr. Usui* by Frank Arjava Petter (translated by Christine M. Grimm), Lotus Press, Twin Lakes/WI, 1998, pg. 13.

16 *The Reiki Sourcebook* by Bronwen and Frans Stiene, O Books, Winchester/UK, New York/USA, 2003, pg. 107.

17 The complete text of these "Questions and Answers" is in *Reiki—The Legacy of Dr. Usui* by Frank Arjava Petter (translated by Christine M. Grimm), Lotus Press, Twin Lakes/WI, 1998, pg. 14-20.

18 *The Reiki Sourcebook* by Bronwen and Frans Stiene, O Books, Winchester/UK, New York/USA, 2003, pg. 108.

19 *Reiki—The Legacy of Dr. Usui* by Frank Arjava Petter (translated by Christine M. Grimm), Lotus Press, Twin Lakes/WI, 1998, pg. 14.

20 Ibid., pg. 20.

21 Ibid., pg. 17.

22 *The Original Reiki Handbook of Dr. Mikao Usui*, edited by Frank Arjava Petter, Lotus Press, Twin Lakes/WI, 2000, pg. 25.

23 Ibid., pg. 29 and *The Reiki Sourcebook* by Bronwen and Frans Stiene, O Books, Winchester/UK, New York/USA, 2003, pg. 110.

24 *The Original Reiki Handbook of Dr. Mikao Usui*, edited by Frank Arjava Petter, Lotus Press, Twin Lakes/WI, 2000, pg. 5.

25 *The Reiki Sourcebook* by Bronwen and Frans Stiene, O Books, Winchester/UK, New York/USA, 2003, pg. 78f.

26 *The Original Reiki Handbook of Dr. Mikao Usui*, edited by Frank Arjava Petter, Lotus Press, Twin Lakes/WI, 2000, pg. 7f and pg. 25.

27 From a German-language article on Reiki in Japan by Hiroko Kasahara, *Reiki Magazin*, Issue 4/2003, pg. 38.

28 Ibid., pg. 41.

29 *The Reiki Sourcebook* by Bronwen and Frans Stiene, O Books, Winchester/UK, New York/USA, 2003, pg. 81.

30 *Reiki—The Legacy of Dr. Usui* by Frank Arjava Petter (translated by Christine M. Grimm), Lotus Press, Twin Lakes/WI, 1998, pg. 19.

31 Telephone conversation with Hiroko Kasahara on August 11, 2004.

32 *The Reiki Sourcebook* by Bronwen and Frans Stiene, O Books, Winchester/UK, New York/USA, 2003, pg. 311

33 From a German-language article on Japanese Poems explained by Hiroko Kasahara, *Reiki Magazin*, Issue 2/2004, pg. 43.

34 *The Spirit of Reiki* by Walter Lübeck, Frank Arjava Petter, and William Lee Rand (translated by Christine M. Grimm), Lotus Press, Twin Lakes/WI, 2002, pg. 290.

35 *The Hayashi Reiki Manual* by Frank Arjava Petter, Tadao Yamaguchi, and Chujiro Hayashi, Lotus Press, Twin Lakes/WI, 2003, pg. 63.

36 *The Reiki Sourcebook* by Bronwen and Frans Stiene, O Books, Winchester/UK, New York/USA, 2003, pg. 80.

37 Ibid.

38 *The Hayashi Reiki Manual* by Frank Arjava Petter, Tadao Yamaguchi, and Chujiro Hayashi, Lotus Press, Twin Lakes/WI, 2003, pg. 5.

39 *The Reiki Sourcebook* by Bronwen and Frans Stiene, O Books, Winchester/UK, New York/USA, 2003, pg. 219.

40 Ibid.

41 Ibid., pg. 125.

42 German-language article on Reiki in Japan by Hiroko Kasahara, *Reiki Magazin*, Issue 4/2003, pg. 40.

43 "Reiki Ryoho—The Art of Conscious Touch" by Frank Arjava Petter, *Reiki News Magazine*, Summer 2004, pg. 46.

44 "Mrs. Takata's Masters. A series of conversations with Reiki Masters initiated by Hawayo Takata. Fran Brown: Storyteller" by Fran Brown, *Reiki Magazine International*, Issue 9, (Feb./March 2001), pg. 21.

45 It is considered certain that Chiyoko Yamaguchi was initiated into the First and Second Degree (*Shoden* and *Okuden*) by Dr. Hayashi within the scope of one(!) five-day seminar (see *The Hayashi Reiki Manual*, pg. 15f.); however, it is unclear whether Dr. Hayashi also initiated her into the Third Degree (*Shinpiden*): Frank Arjava Petter writes: "Chiyoko-Sensei, as her students tenderly called her, was trained as a Reiki Teacher in 1939, as an 18-year-old, by Dr. Hayashi." (See German-language article on Chiyoko Yamaguchi: "A Life on the Reiki Path" by Frank Arjava Petter, *Reiki Magazin*, Issue 1/2004, pg. 44.) Bronwen and Frans Stiene write that according to information from Hyakuten Inamoto, who was trained in Reiki by Chiyoko Yamaguchi before she officially called her system *Jikiden Reiki*: "It appears she never learnt to become an official teacher but was taught the attunement from a relative who was hosting a course for Chujiro Hayashi. (…). (…) she did not officially study to become a teacher." (*The Reiki Sourcebook*, pg. 125 and pg. 262).

46 From a German-language article on Chiyoko Yamaguchi: "A Life on the Reiki Path" by Frank Arjava Petter, *Reiki Magazin*, Issue 1/2004, pg. 45.

47 *The Hayashi Reiki Manual* by Frank Arjava Petter, Tadao Yamaguchi, and Chujiro Hayashi, Lotus Press, Twin Lakes/WI, 2003, pg. 7f.

48 Ibid., pg. 9

49 From text material on Hiroshi Doi that Hiroko Kasahara was kind enough to send me.

50 Ibid.

51 Ibid.

52 Ibid., as well as *Iyashino Gendai Reiki-ho*—Modern REIKI METHOD for Healing by Hiroshi Doi, Fraser Journal Publishing, Coquitlam, British Columbia, 2000, pg. 205.

53 Ibid., Also see an article on *Gendai Reiki Ho* by Hiroshi Doi, published in German language in *Reiki Magazin*, Issue 3/2003, pg. 21.

54 From text material on Hiroshi Doi that Hiroko Kasahara was kind enough to send me.

55 *The Reiki Sourcebook* by Bronwen and Frans Stiene, O Books, Winchester/UK, New York/USA, 2003, pg. 130.

56 From an article on *Gendai Reiki Ho* by Hiroshi Doi, published in German language in *Reiki Magazin*, Issue 3/2003, pg. 20.

57 From text material on Hiroshi Doi that Hiroko Kasahara was kind enough to send me.

58 From an article on *Gendai Reiki Ho* by Hiroshi Doi, published in German language in *Reiki Magazin*, Issue 3/2003, pg. 22.

59 Ibid.

60 Ibid., pg. 23.

61 Ibid.

62 Ibid.

63 Ibid.

64 Ibid.

65 Ibid.

66 Ibid., pg. 22f.

67 Ibid., pg. 22.

68 Ibid., pg. 22 / The information on the dates comes from *The Spirit of Reiki* by Walter Lübeck, Frank Arjava Petter, and William Lee Rand (translated by Christine M. Grimm), Lotus Press, Twin Lakes/WI, 2002, pg. 17.

69 *Iyashino Gendai Reiki-ho*—Modern REIKI METHOD for Healing by Hiroshi Doi, Fraser Journal Publishing, Coquitlam, British Columbia, 2000, pg. 79.

70 Ibid., pg. 194

71 Ibid.

72 "An Interview with Hiroshi Doi—Part ll" by William Lee Rand, *Reiki News Magazine*, Fall 2003, pg. 13.

73 Ibid.

74 All of the information in this paragraph is from: "An Interview with Hiroshi Doi—Part ll" by William Lee Rand, *Reiki News Magazine*, Fall 2003, pg. 13.

75 *The Spirit of Reiki* by Walter Lübeck, Frank Arjava Petter, and William Lee Rand (translated by Christine M. Grimm), Lotus Press, Twin Lakes/WI, 2002, pg. 37.

76 *Reiki—Best Practices* by Walter Lübeck and Frank Arjava Petter, Lotus Press, Twin Lakes/WI, 2003, in: "What is a Technique?" by Frank Arjava Petter, pg. 9.

Chapter 7: New Paths

1   Conversation with Phyllis Furumoto in June 2004 in Idaho.

2   Ibid.

3   Ibid.

4   Ibid.

5   Ibid.

6   From a German-language article on Reiki: "Traditional and Modern" by Oliver Klatt, *Reiki Magazin*, Issue 3/2001, pg. 38.

7   Ibid.

8   From the article: "From Hawayo Takata to the Present" by Paul Mitchell, published in German language in DAO Reiki Special Edition 2, August 1996, pg. 14.

9   Observations from my own experience in relation to my years of working as the editor-in-chief of the German-language *Reiki Magazin*.

10 Ibid.

11 From a German-language article on Reiki and Money: "Energy in Exchange" by Oliver Klatt, *Reiki Magazin*, Issue 2/2002.

12 *Reiki—Best Practices* by Walter Lübeck and Frank Arjava Petter, Lotus Press, Twin Lakes/WI, 2003, text by Walter Lübeck, pg. 37.

13 *The Power of Reiki. An Ancient Hands-on Healing Technique* by Tanmaya Honervogt, Henry Holt and Company, New York 1998 / Reprint with friendly permission of the author and the German publisher, Innenwelt Verlag, Cologne, Germany.

14 From a German-language article on "The Life Path with Reiki" by Walter Lübeck and Frank Arjava Petter, *Reiki Magazin* Special Edition, in cooperation with the Windpferd publishing company, Berlin 2002, pg. 4.

15 This text is written on the basis of different main sources about the Bach Flower Therapy.

16 *Das Reiki-Buch. Heilung und Weg* by Ute Wehrend (German-language book), Arche Noah Verlag, Oster-Schnatebüll, 2000, pg. 126 / Translated by Christine M. Grimm.

17 *Aura-Soma, Bach-Blueten und Reiki* by Anita Bind-Klinger (German-language book), Aquamarin Verlag, Grafing, 1998.

18 This text is written on the basis of different main sources about Aura-Soma.

19 *Aura-Soma, Bach-Blueten und Reiki* by Anita Bind-Klinger (German-language book), Aquamarin Verlag, Grafing, 1998.

20 This text is written on the basis of different main sources about gemstones.

21 Minerals = the mineral components of plant and animal organisms that remain after burning body substances into ash.

22 *Esoterische Therapien* by Dietmar Krämer (German-language book), Ansata Verlag, Interlaken/Switzerland. From the German-language website: www. esoterik-forum.de/esoterik-woerterbuch/edelsteintherapie.htm (April 2001).

23 *Reiki with Gemstones* by Ursula Klinger-Raatz (now: Klinger-Omenka), translated by Christine M. Grimm, Lotus Press, Twin Lakes/WI, 1997.

24 From a German-language interview with Ursula Klinger-Omenka on Reiki with Gemstones by Jürgen Kindler, *Reiki Magazin*, Issue 1/2001, pg. 15f. (Quote translated by Christine M. Grimm. Slight language-related changes were made to the original excerpt by the editor.)

25 This text is written on the basis of different main sources about the chakra theories.

26 In response to my question as whether it is true according to his knowledge that Mrs. Takata did not teach any chakra work in her courses, Paul Mitchell wrote in an e-mail (7/16/04): "It is true that Mrs. Takata did not ever mention the chakras as part of the treatment. I imagine if you asked her about it outside the class after practicing for a while, she would say that of course the chakras are affected by the treatment. She did not focus any of the treatment on the chakras or mention them."

27 This text is written on the basis of different main sources about working with sound.

28 *Nada Brahma—Die Welt ist Klang* by Joachim-Ernst Berendt (German-language book), Rowohlt Taschenbuch Verlag, Hamburg, 1985, pg. 39 / Translated by Christine M. Grimm.

29 From a German-language interview with Peter Stein on Reiki and Sound by Oliver Klatt, *Reiki Magazin*, Issue 4/2003, pg. 10.

30 *Letters to the Schools*, Volume 2, 1 November 1982 by J. Krishnamurti, Copyright: Krishnamurti Foundation Trust / Thanks to Bernd Hollstein from the Krishnamurti-Forum, Germany, who kindly sent this quote to me.

31 From a German-language article on The Fire Bird by Kristina Mascher, *Reiki Magazin*, Issue 3/2004, pg. 47.

32 *Reiki—Best Practices* by Walter Lübeck and Frank Arjava Petter, Lotus Press, Twin Lakes/WI, 2003, in: "What is a Technique?" by Frank Arjava Petter, pg. 52.

33 From a German-language article about the inscription on the memorial stone for Mikao Usui (in the translation from Japanese by Hiroko Kasahara), *Reiki Magazin*, Issue 2/2003, pg. 40.

34 From an interview with Paul Mitchell on *Usui Shiki Ryoho*, Part 1, by Oliver Klatt, published in German language in *Reiki Magazin*, Issue 2/2004, pg. 38f / For the interview in English language see the website: www.reiki-magazin.de, keyword "International", scroll down to: "Usui Shiki Ryoho"—an interview with Paul David Mitchell, October 2003.

35 *Nada Brahma—Die Welt ist Klang* by Joachim-Ernst Berendt (German-language book), Rowohlt Taschenbuch Verlag, Hamburg, 1985, pg. 39 / Translated by Christine M. Grimm.

36 From text material on her healing work with sounds that Dagmar Fröhlich was kind enough to send me.

37 Ibid.

38 Ibid.

39 In addition to the text for the exercise, the idea for drawing 2 (Cycle of the Water) also came from Dagmar Fröhlich.

Chapter 8: Transcendence

1 Transcendence = crossing the boundaries of experience and what can be recognized with the senses.

2 This text is written on the basis of different main sources about channeling as well as personal observations and conversations with Sabine Fennell.

3 From a German-language article on Channeling: "Mit Sonnenkraft im Herzen" by Sabine Fennell, *Reiki Magazin*, Issue 2/2004, pg. 31.

4 From written material that Sabine Fennell was kind enough to give me.

5 ARD = Main television station in Germany

6 From a German-language article on Miracles through Spiritual Healing by Christian Stippekohl, *Reiki Magazin*, Issue 1/2004, pg. 21 / The excerpt was slightly adapted to reflect the original text by Christian Stippekohl.

7 I received the information contained in this paragraph from Anne Hübner during a telephone conversation on August 3, 2004.

8 Ibid.

9 This text is written on the basis of different main sources about Buddhism.

10 From an issue of *KursKontakte* (German-language magazine), 2003.

11 *Weltreligionen—Weltfrieden—Weltethos*, German-language brochure by the foundation *Weltethos fuer interkulturelle und interreligioese Forschung, Bildung, Begegnung*, Tübingen, 2000, pg. 11 / Translated by Christine M. Grimm.

12 Ibid.

13 "Mrs. Takata Opens Minds to Reiki," *Reiki Magazine International,* Issue 2 (Dec. 1999/Jan. 2000): "Before she continues her story, Mrs. Takata explains that Reiki was already mentioned in the ancient history of Japan and that the Buddhist Sutras, the sacred scriptures, refer to it. Reiki dates back at least 2,500 years." Excerpt from: San Mateo Times, May 17, 1975 / "We Are All Healers" by Sally Hammond, *Reiki Magazine International,* Issue 1 (Oct./Nov. 1999): "The Usui System is a method that Usui revived according to the Buddhist sacred scriptures, a path of attunement into Reiki (…)." Excerpt from: *We are all Healers* by Sally Hammond, Ballantine Books, 1973.

14 "Experience of a Buddha-Reiki Connection" by Ray Pine, *Reiki Magazine International,* Issue 14 (Dec. 2001/Jan. 2002), pg. 9 / The article also includes photos of the described depictions.

15 Rainbow Reiki by Walter Lübeck (German-language book), Windpferd Verlag, Aitrang, 2002, pg. 13f / Translated by Christine M. Grimm

16 From an interview with Swam Prem Jagran on Peace Practice by Oliver Klatt, *Reiki Magazin,* Issue 1/2004, pg. 29 / Originally translated from Italian by Benedetta Grossrubatscher.

17 *Das neue Lexikon der Esoterik* by Marc Roberts (German-language version), Goldmann Verlag, Munich, 1995, pg. 429.

18 From an interview with Swam Prem Jagran on Peace Practice by Oliver Klatt, *Reiki Magazin,* Issue 1/2004, pg. 28 / Originally translated from Italian by Benedetta Grossrubatscher.

19 *Das neue Lexikon der Esoterik* by Marc Roberts (German-language version), Goldmann Verlag, Munich, 1995, pg. 430 (Tantrism), pg. 456 (Yantra), pg. 145 (Bija), and pg. 380 (Mudra).

20 *Buddhistische Persoenlichkeiten* by Erdmute Klein (German-language book), Goldmann Verlag, Munich, 1998, pg. 183.

21 The information in this paragraph comes from written material that Swami Prem Jagran was kind enough to give me, as well as from the interview with Swami Prem Jagran on Practicing Peace by Oliver Klatt, *Reiki Magazin,* Issue 1/2004, pg. 28 / Lama = Tibetan-Buddhist teacher, master, or sage; Tulku = one who allows himself to be consciously reincarnated for the benefit of all sentient beings. He manifests to make it possible for beings to access their Buddha nature. (…) Tulku (Tibetan) means "illusion body"; Rinpoche = "precious master." Honorary title for high-ranking lamas or scholars (from: *Buddhistische Persoenlichkeiten* by Erdmute Klein (German-language book), Goldmann Verlag, Munich, 1998, pg. 181f.)

22 From an interview with Swam Prem Jagran on Peace Practice by Oliver Klatt, *Reiki Magazin,* Issue 1/2004, pg. 27 / Originally translated from Italian by Benedetta Grossrubatscher.

23 Ibid., pg. 29 / For reasons of clarity, the quote was changed at one point (*Ngal So Chag Wang Reiki* instead of Reiki), with friendly permission of Swami Prem Jagran.

24 Personal observations and a conversation with Swami Prem Jagran on August 13, 2004.

25 Quote from written material that Swami Prem Jagran was kind enough to give me (text by Swami Prem Jagran, July 2004, Verona, Italy).

26 Ibid.
27 Ibid.
28 Ibid.
29 Ibid.
30 From a previously unpublished interview with Swami Prem Jagran on The Fragrance of Emptiness by Oliver Klatt, November 2003, Berlin / Quote translated by Christine M. Grimm.
31 The information in this paragraph comes from written material that Swami Prem Jagran was kind enough to give me.

Chapter 9: Spirituality

1 "The Wheel of Reiki" by Phyllis Furumoto, Reiki Info (former Swiss Reiki Magazine), Issue 1/1995, pg. 7, as well as an interview with Paul Mitchell on the Usui Shiki Ryoho, Part 2, by Oliver Klatt, published in German language in Reiki Magazin, Issue 3/2004, pg. 38f (For the interview in English language see the website: www.reiki-magazin.de, keyword "International", scroll down to: "Usui Shiki Ryoho"—an interview with Paul David Mitchell, October 2003.)
2 Lexikon der Esoterik by Werner Bogun and Norbert Strät (German-language book), Falken, Cologne, 1997, pg. 636.
3 Esoterik by Antoine Faivre (German-language version), Aurum Verlag, Edition Roter Löwe, Braunschweig, 1996, pg. 13.
4 Seen in this way, it also makes sense that one of the basic principles of teachings and system with an esoteric orientation must be to not immediately reveal everything at the beginning that is significant within this context but disclose the corresponding contents step-by-step.
5 Projekt Menschwerdung by Gerd-Christian Weniger (German-language book), Spektrum—Akademischer Verlag, Berlin, 2003, pg. 83.
6 Ernst Benz, an expert on the history of religion, quoted in Zu Gast bei den Religionen der Welt by Monika Tworuschka, Herder spektrum, Freiburg im Breisgau, 2000, pg. 170.
7 Ibid., Zen Poem, translated by Christine M. Grimm
8 H.H. The Dalai Lama in What Is Enlightenment?, Issue 22, Spring/Summer 2002, pg. 131

Chapter 10: Healing

1 "Reiki—Review of a Biofield Therapy. History, Theory, Practice, and Research" by Pamela Miles and Gala True, Alternative Therapies in Health and Medicine, Vol. 9, No. 2, March/April 2003, pg. 62-72, www.alternative-therapies.com / The article is available at Pamela Miles' website: www.pamelamilesreiki.com, keyword: "References and Resources", then: Articles.
2 "Reiki—Review of a Biofield Therapy. Interview with Pamela Miles" by Barbara McDaniel, Reiki Magazine International, Issue 24 (Aug./Sept. 2003), pg. 26.
3 The Spirit of Reiki by Walter Lübeck, Frank Arjava Petter, and William Lee Rand (translated by Christine M. Grimm), Lotus Press, Twin Lakes/WI, 2002, pg. 271.

4 "Reiki—Review of a Biofield Therapy. Interview with Pamela Miles" by Barbara McDaniel, *Reiki Magazine International*, Issue 24 (Aug./Sept. 2003), pg. 26.

5 *Return of the Rishi—A Doctor's Search for the Ultimate Healer* by Deepak Chopra, M.D., Houghton Mifflin Company, Boston 1988, pg. 83.

6 *Der Heilende Buddha* by Raoul Birnbaum (German-language version), Gondrom Verlag, Bindlach, 1990, pg. 37 / Translated by Christine M. Grimm.

7 *Projekt Menschwerdung* by Gerd-Christian Weniger (German-language book), Spektrum—Akademischer Verlag, Berlin, 2003, pg. 120 / Translated by Christine M. Grimm.

Address Section
with Information on the Contributors

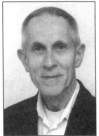

Don Alexander

E-Mail: donalex.1@email.com
Website: www.Heart-of-Reiki.com
Tel.: Not provided

Don Alexander, Buddhist monk in Thailand from 1968-77, teaches "Heart of Reiki" and "Mystic Heart of Reiki" seminars to enrich the practice of Reiki students of all levels. His book *The Mystic Heart of Reiki* and his seminars are enlivened by his own experience with Buddhist stories and practical wisdom from Japan.

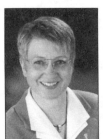

Anita Bind-Klinger

E-Mail: anita.bind@arcor.de
Website: Not provided
Tel.: ++49-6071-21434 (Germany)

Anita Bind-Klinger, born in 1954, is a naturopath, Reiki Master, cosmo-energeticist, and author of several books. She has been working in her own practice in Dieburg, Germany since 1988, showing people holistic perspectives and providing guidance through classical homeopathy, Reiki (since 1985), gemstones, Bach Flowers, and Aura-Soma essences in individual sessions. Her German-language books, including *Aura-Soma, Bach-Blueten und Reiki*, have been published by the *Aquamarin-Verlag*.

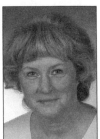

Sabine Fennell

E-Mail: SabineFennell@t-online.de
Website: www.sabine-fennell.privat.t-online.de
Tel.: ++49-3322-213291 (Germany)

Sabine Fennell, born in 1948, is a former elementary school teacher and has been a Reiki Master/Teacher since 1992. She is a medium, healer, and writer of books on cosmic healing and spiritual poetry. She has been a channeler since 1996 and is especially in very tangible contact with spiritual teachers in the light. She offers channeling sessions, medial training, and consultations on fulfilling your life plan, calling, self-healing, and happy relationships.

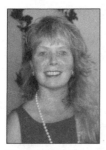

Dagmar Fröhlich

E-Mail: info@klangraum-dagmar-froehlich.de
Website: www.klangraum-dagmar-froehlich.de
Tel.: ++49-611-6900639 (Germany)

Dagmar Fröhlich, born in 1955, is a certified educator, psycho-organic body therapist (Paul Boyesen), company trainer, and coach. She has been a Reiki Master/Teacher since 1993 of the sixth generation, The Reiki Alliance, offering First and Second Degree, qualified Master/ Teacher training and spiritual therapy with Reiki. Her areas of specialty are: prenatal and early disorders, abuse. Also performs transformational work, as well as therapy and concerts with healing primal sounds.

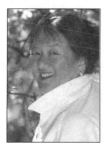

Phyllis Lei Furumoto

E-Mail: usuireiki@mac.com
Website: www.usuireiki-ogm.com
Tel.: 208-6829009 (USA)

Many people recognize Phyllis Lei Furumoto as the Lineage Bearer of *Usui Shiki Ryoho*, after the death of Takata Sensei in 1980. Since this time, she has been functioning as the spiritual head, as well as a devoted student, of this practice. She brings to her work a passion for supporting spiritual community and furthering individual personal development.

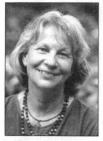

Himani—H. Gerber

E-Mail: info@OshoNeoReiki.com
Website: www.OshoNeoReiki.com
Tel.: ++351-96-8450584 (Portugal)

Himani has been practicing Reiki since 1982. For many years, she taught at the International Osho Multiversity/India, in Europe, and on Taiwan. She gives initiations throughout the world, trainings in metaphysical energy work, and exhibitions of her paintings on inner Feng Shui. In 1996, she founded the *Osho Institute of Neo-Reiki and Creativity*.

343

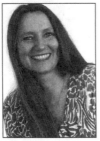

Tanmaya Honervogt

E-Mail: tanmaya@gmx.de
Website: www.school-of-usui-reiki.com
Tel.: ++44-1769-580899 (England)

Tanmaya Honervogt is a Reiki Master and book author. Her bestseller *The Power of Reiki. An Ancient Hands-on Healing Technique* (England: *Reiki—Healing and Harmony through the Hands*) has been published in 18 languages up to now. Tanmaya has been practicing Reiki for the past 21 years. In 1995, she established the *School of Usui Reiki* in Devon/England. She holds seminars and lectures in Europe, Japan, and the USA.

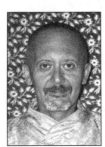

Swami Prem Jagran

E-Mail: info@jagran.it
Website: www.jagran.it
Tel.: ++49-33208-21873 (Germany)

Swami Prem Jagran, healer and Ngal So Chag Wang Reiki® Master, was born in Italy in 1957. Many great lamas and spiritual teachers have recognized that Swami Prem Jagran has the characteristics of a healer and a great sensitivity. People from all stratums of society and from around the world find in Swami Prem Jagran a valid help in their personal search for harmony, inner peace, and both spiritual and psychophysical healing.

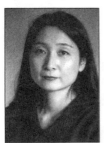

Hiroko Kasahara

E-Mail: Hiroko.kasahara@t-online.de
Website: www.reiki-runen.de
Tel.: ++49-2232-941872 (Germany)

Hiroko Kasahara was born in Tokyo in 1962. She was trained by Hiroshi Doi as a Reiki Master/Teacher of *Gendai Reiki-hô*, whose methods unite Western and Japanese traditional Reiki. She is the First Chairperson of the German Professional Association for Psychosocial Healthcare. Among other things, the goal of this professional association is the development of legal protection for Reiki practitioners and the legalization as a specialized group with a complete professional image.

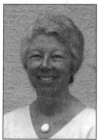

Ursula Klinger-Omenka

E-Mail: post@chidera-edle-steine.com
Website: www.chidera-edle-steine.com
Tel.: ++49-8382-888333 (Germany)

Since 1983, Ursula Klinger-Omenka has been treating clients with Reiki in her own practice, often in cooperation with doctors. She is a Reiki Master (initiated in 1988 by Phyllis Furumoto) and author of books such as *Reiki with Gemstones* (Lotus Press), holds seminars, and gives consultations. Several long visits to Nigeria, where she built a Reiki clinic together with her husband, opened up new paths of humanity and spirituality for her.

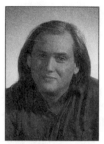

Walter Lübeck

E-Mail: info@rainbowreiki.net
Website: www.rainbowreiki.net
Tel.: ++49-5154-970040 (Germany)

Walter Lübeck works as an international spiritual teacher and book author. He has developed his Rainbow Reiki System on the basis of traditional Reiki according to Dr. Mikao Usui since 1989. With his work, Walter would like to make a contribution toward the quickest possible beginning of a new Golden Age for all being on the earth.

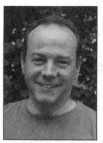

Peter Mascher

E-Mail: reikiprocess@yahoo.de
Website: www.reikiprocess.com
Tel.: ++32-3-2395598 (Belgium)

Peter Mascher is a professional instrumentalist (viola), singer (baritone), and Reiki Master. He was initiated by Don Alexander and teaches "Heart of Reiki" seminars on the *Shoden* level (First Degree) together with him. With a creative approach, he teaches Ki exercises, Process Work, meditation, and free improvisation in various Reiki communities, as well as at home in Antwerp, Belgium. He is currently writing a book on Reiki energy, Japan, and the sacred mountains.

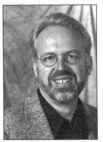

Paul Mitchell

E-Mail: pauldm@earthlink.net
Website: www.usuireiki-ogm.com
Tel.: 208-6824427 (USA)

Paul Mitchell has been practicing Reiki since 1978 and was a student of Mrs. Takata. He is one of the 22 masters trained by Mrs. Takata to carry on her work of practicing and teaching *Usui Shiki Ryoho*. He has been invited to 21 countries worldwide to facilitate classes, workshops, and retreats for Reiki students.

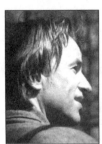

Frank Arjava Petter

E-Mail: Arjava@ReikiDharma.com
Website: www.ReikiDharma.com
Tel.: ++49-211-5073810 (Germany)

Frank Arjava Petter is well-known and esteemed in the international Reiki family for his work of clarification. His books, published by Lotus Press, have already been translated into 16 languages and have become international bestsellers. After a long stay abroad, Arjava has been living in Düsseldorf, Germany, with his companion in life since the end of 2002.

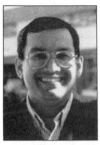

Dr. Ranga J. Premaratna, Ph.D

E-Mail: ranga1@bigpond.com
Website: www.reikijinkeido.com.au
Tel.: ++61-2-99693920 (Australia)

Dr. Ranga J. Premaratna received his BSc., MSc., and Ph.D degrees in Food and Nutritional Science. He received complete training in Reiki and the EnerSense (Buddho) System of Natural Healing from Ven. Seiji Takamori in 1990 while working at the University of Wisconsin, Food Research Institute, as a post-doctoral research scientist. Ranga teaches *Reiki Jin Kei Do* stages 1 to Master, as well as the *EnerSense* (Buddho) System of Healing, in Sydney, Australia.

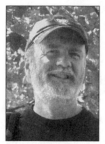

William Lee Rand

E-Mail: center@reiki.org
Website: www.reiki.org
Tel.: 248-9488112 (USA)

William Lee Rand is the founder of *The International Center for Reiki Training*. The Center is dedicated to helping all Reiki people worldwide improve their Reiki practice. Its website has 350 pages and offers 150 free articles, free downloads, a web store, and many other services and features.

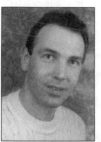

Edwin Zimmerli

E-Mail: edwin.zimmerli@starcon.ch
Website: www.starcon.ch
Tel.: ++41-44-7901669 (Switzerland)

Edwin Zimmerli, born in 1960, has been a Master/ Teacher of Reiki and *Rei-Ki Balancing*® since 1995. Since this time, he has specialized in energy and light work for supporting the lightbody processes. He works with bipolar energy attunements (connection with the new earth and reconnection with the cosmic meridians) and directs the *Starcon Lightbody* seminar in Uetikon on Lake Zurich, Switzerland. He is currently working on a book titled: *Die Reiki-Kraft im Lichtkoerper-Prozess* (The Reiki Power in the Lightbody Process).

Acknowledgements

I would first like to thank Jürgen Kindler for the extensive support that he has given me for many years in the editorial work for *Reiki Magazin*, as well as in my personal development as a Reiki Master. This book ultimately grew out of my work for *Reiki Magazin*, and Jürgen supported this project right from the start. I would like to thank him for his valuable feedback and the many hours of discussions and reflections.

I would also like to express my profound gratitude to Paul Mitchell for his loving wisdom, continuous presence, and his support of my path with Reiki. I would also like to thank Swami Prem Jagran for the many important insights and the healing that came to me through him.

My deepest thanks also goes to Phyllis Lei Furumoto, Wanja Twan, Sabine Fennell, and Don Alexander, from whom I was able to learn much, as well as to Peter Mascher, Hiroko Kasahara, Walter Lübeck and Frank Arjava Petter for the sharing that has always been inspiring.

Furthermore, I thank Simone Grashoff and Frank Doerr for the many years of good cooperation in the area of Reiki, as well as for the many personal encounters.

My special thanks goes to Janine Warmbier for creating the drawings in this book and for the many years of creative work for *Reiki Magazin*. Annett Landmann also deserves special thanks for the help in producing the photos that served as the models for the drawings in this book, as well as Simone von Mach.

I would like to express my very special thanks to my beloved companion in life Heidrun Goslowsky for her constant helpful feedback after the first proofreading of my texts. Without her support and openness, this book, as well as the overall circumstances of my work in relation to Reiki, would not have been possible in the current form.

I would also like to thank Monika Jünemann of the *Windpferd Verlag* in Germany for the helpful support during the beginning phase of the book, as well as for the ongoing inspiring conversations.

My special thanks also goes to Werner Plötz and Gegs Zimmermann, from whom I learned the craft of creating a book as complex as this during my early professional years.

I thank all of the authors and Reiki Master colleagues who have contributed an exercise or a text to this book.

And finally, I thank everyone who has written about the Usui System of Reiki during the past 25 years—this has made it possible for me to compile such an extensive and complex work.

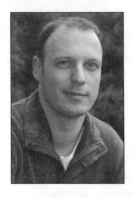

About the Author

Oliver Klatt, born in 1967, has practiced the Usui System of Reiki since 1994. He passes on the knowledge that he has acquired over many years as a Reiki Master in his Reiki seminars, as well as in his activities as a book author and lecturer.

He received a Master of Arts Degree upon concluding his studies in journalism, film, and television at the *Freie Universität Berlin* and worked as an editor and project head.

In 2000, he received the initiation into the Master Degree of the Usui System of Reiki Healing from Paul David Mitchell, one of the 22 Reiki Masters who were trained by Hawayo Takata. Oliver Klatt's many years of training were marked by intensive personal development and a lively exchange with Masters and students throughout the world.

Since 2001 he has worked in Berlin and all of Germany as a Reiki Teacher and lecturer. In addition, he serves as the editor-in-chief of the German-language *Reiki Magazin.*

Information on Reiki Seminars and treatments with Oliver Klatt:

Oliver Klatt
Hildegardstr. 25A, 10715 Berlin, Germany
Phone: ++49-(0)30-85731646
Fax: ++49-(0)30-85731644
E-Mail: info@epanoui.de
www.epanoui.de

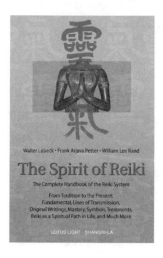

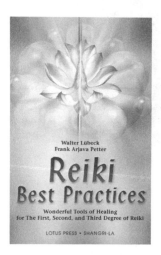

W. Lübeck · F. A. Petter · W. L. Rand
The Spirit of Reiki
The Complete Handbook of the Reiki System · From Tradition to the Present: Fundamental, Lines of Transmission, Original Writings, Mastery, Symbols, Treatments, Reiki as a Spiritual Path in Life, and Much More

Never before, have three Reiki masters from different lineages and with extensive background come together to share their experience.

A wealth of information on Reiki for the first time brought together in one place. The broad spectrum of topics range from the search for a scientific explanation of Reiki energy to Reiki as a spiritual path. It also includes the understanding of Dr. Usui's original healing methods, how Reiki is currently practiced in Japan, an analysis of the Western evolution of Reiki, and a discussion about the direction Reiki is likely to take in the future.

312 pages · $19.95
150 photos and b/w illustrations
ISBN 0-914955-67-5

Walter Lübeck · Frank Arjava Petter
Reiki – Best Practices
Wonderful Tools of Healing for the First, Second and Third Degree of Reiki

Western Reiki techniques, published and presented in great detail for the first time

The internationally renowned Reiki Masters Walter Lübeck and Frank Arjava Petter introduce primarily Western Reiki techniques and place a valuable tool in the hands of every Reiki practitioner for applying Reiki in a specific and effective way for protection and healing.

A total of 60 techniques, such as: aura massage with Reiki, de-programming of old patterns, karma clearing, protecting against energy loss, Tantra with Reiki are exclusively presented and described in detail for the first time in this fascinating guide.

296 pages · $19.95
richly illustrated with many b/w drawings
ISBN 0-914955-74-8

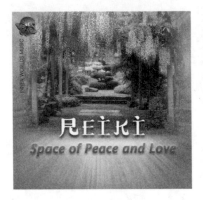

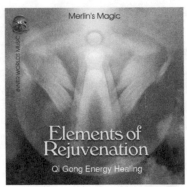

Merlin's Magic
Reiki –
Space of Peace and Love

This is the most meditative Merlin's Magic production up to now, with compositions uniting in the "silent eye" of Reiki. The sounds of Far Eastern spheres unfold in virtual deep stillness, led by the rhythm of the heart. 60 minutes of complete melodic pleasure, suitable for all Reiki techniques. Accompanied by a small booklet of 16 pages, written by the world-renowned Reiki teacher and best-selling author, Frank Arjava Petter. Andreas Mock, whose unique style of gently flowing melodies and meditative magic is splendidly supported by various outstanding musicians, always enjoys creating music in cooperation with distinguished experts from a variety of healing modalities.

60 minute CD · $16.95
ISBN: 0-910261-25-3

Merlin's Magic
Elements of Rejuvenation

The sounds of Tao. Perfectly accentuated harmonies allow you to immerse in the Far Eastern enchantment of an eternal fountain of youth and charge yourself with fresh qi energy. For thousands of years, Taoists have researched unflaggingly and enlarged humanity's knowledge about prolonging life and increasing mental powers. Qigong exercises enable you to use your existing qi in an optimal manner. The result are astonishing abilities to heal yourself and others.

Together with two excellent qigong masters, the renowned group Merlin's Magic, led by Andreas Mock, has wonderfully translated the energy of qigong into the dimension of a fascinating and energizing world of sounds.

60-minute CD · $17.95
with a 16-pages booklet
ISBN: 0-910261-43-1